LOW

THE 7 WAYS YOU CAN DEAL WITH DEPRESSION

CYRUS BROWN

CONTENTS

INTRODUCTION

"Once you choose hope, anything is possible."

— CHRISTOPHER REEVE

From as far back as we can remember, we have been living a life that is a constant journey from one point to the next. We were told to grow up when we were kids, and to get a job when we were teenagers. We are told to work hard now so that we can get all we want in life later. We are told to work smart, not hard, to get ahead of everyone else.

We firmly believe that this is life as we know it, so we keep pushing ourselves and taking on too much, more than we can handle. We readily take on more stress to keep us alert, motivated, and ready to respond when needed. It could be a work deadline or a high-stakes sports game. We wouldn't be ready and primed to attack were it not for taking in all that stress. But, over time, that stress can actually lead to an enemy we are ill-equipped to handle: depression.

What causes stress? Anything and everything. Even the happiest moments, such as getting married, can have you in a constant state of worry, especially if there aren't enough hors d'oeuvres. Even starting a brand new job or career can have you concerned about what kind of impression you are about to make. In short, nothing is sacred in front of depression. No one is safe. Not even you.

Especially not you. That's why you are here, isn't it?

Whether it is because you are suffering from depression, and have been for a long time, or you are worried about becoming depressed in the future, you know that there is something you need to do in your life. You can see that the path of ups and downs that you are on is nothing but a hamster wheel that you constantly run on with absolutely no rewards and no happiness associated with it. You know that there is a better life out there; a life where you no longer have to be tense and tightly wound up every time you are asked to do something. A life where you have the self-assurance to say no when you need to. In short, you are looking to feel empowered, and take the reins of your life to lead in the direction you want.

And if it isn't you, then it may be someone you know. Someone who is near and dear to you, whose place in your life is invaluable. Someone who you see suffering from depression but who hasn't come to terms with their circumstances yet. Someone you know needs help and should have a normal life again, where they have better control over their emotions and relationships. And you feel like you can help them a great deal by being their guide and helping them follow a holistic path that isn't riddled with antidepressants and medications that will leave them in a drug-filled haze.

If that someone is you, you want to be free from the overwhelming cloud of depression for good.

Low – The 7 Ways You Can Deal With Depression is a step-by-step guide that aims to help people with symptoms of depression break out of the cycle of darkness that keeps them periodically low and socially withdrawn, losing friendships because they cannot cope with their circumstances. It helps people to recognize how their unhealthy lifestyle choices may be responsible for keeping them in a state of anxiety and despair, and that they need to rediscover their zest for life.

This book focuses on how our environment can be used to enrich and nourish us, or it can be used to keep us in the dark. Whether it is because of a lack of motivation or energy or being cooped up at home with TV and smartphones, it will illustrate just how these negative habits continue to debilitate us and diminish our interest in our own well-being. It also focuses on finding our sources of energy and what motivates us to get out of bed every morning so that we endeavor to become the best versions of ourselves against the never-ending torrent of depressive situations this modern world throws at us.

Each of the chapters within provide a detailed understanding of the different problems and situations we face, and how best to navigate through them. It could be due to the stress we endure from living in a fast-paced and dynamic environment, or the food that we eat and the medications we use to nourish our lives. It could be understanding the role of our environment and nature in our lives, or how technology disrupts the natural flow and nourishment that our bodies require. And it could also be the role of having a clear mind and concentration, as well as being involved with friends and activities that continue to enrich us spiritually.

Born in New Jersey and later having moved to New York City to study medicine, Cyrus Brown has spent several years enhancing his knowledge about Natural Medicine and wholesome practices for improving human biology and finding easy and practical methods to bring the body back to an optimal balance. From his time in San Diego to travelling to India to gain a deeper understanding of Ayurvedic medicine, Brown is an ardent believer in the bounties of nature and their power to influence our physiology for the better. Whether it is our physical, emotional, or mental health, Brown's innate understanding of our body's responses to natural and medicinal treatments makes Low – The 7 Ways You Can Deal With Depression the perfect guide to achieve spiritual freedom.

With five years of studying medicine and Ayurveda, and another three years spent in a Himalayan temple in the company of monks, Brown's expertise and knowledge can help you achieve balance in your emotional state. Furthermore, his insights also come from first-hand experience as the techniques he focuses on are the same ones that helped him to overcome his own battle against depression and rebuild a balanced life. No one can understand the gravity and severity of an issue such as depression more than he can, and his passion and empathy in helping people to achieve freedom from its hold over our lives is why he has endeavored to present his expertise in this book.

With thorough and well-researched scientific information about the causes of depression and the natural solutions that are often overlooked, Low – The 7 Ways You Can Deal With Depression takes you to the heart of the matter by showing you how depression affects you on a physiological level. By helping you to gain a detailed understanding of what has ailed you for so long, you will then be able to understand and counteract each of these symptoms with your very own precision tools that are both natural and holistic.

You will truly be at one with nature and let it provide you with the healthy means to achieve a balanced lifestyle that can easily fight depression for the long-term.

1

SOCIETY ON A FORMULA ONE RACE

"Sometimes your joy is the source of your smile, but sometimes your smile can be the source of your joy."

— THICH NHAT HANH

Welcome to life! It's glamorous, it's glitzy, it's vibrant, and you will meet people from numerous backgrounds and preferences. Some you will love instantly, some you will never want to see again, and some will be constants in your life as the days go by. You will have expectations from others and for others. And in the pursuit of fulfilling these expectations or having your own fulfilled, you will undergo a condition that is bound to make your life experiences something that you would rather not be experiencing.

And that, dear reader, is stress.

Surely you have heard of it, and if not, then you must definitely have felt it in one form or another without knowing what it truly was. Even now as you flip through these pages, you must be feeling something welling up inside you that makes you uncomfortable, or a sensation that something is weighing you down and you have no way of shaking off. So it helps to understand exactly what stress is and how it is affecting you.

Simply put, stress is a state of mind that, if left unchecked, can cause a host of mental and physical illnesses. It affects all age and social groups and affects people on various levels including personal, professional, psychosocial, and so on. This is largely because of the normalization of stress as part and parcel of our working lifestyle. Most workplaces, whether they are white-collar or blue-collar, put a lot of pressure on people to fulfill expectations. It could be the expectations of the employer for them to go above and beyond in their work. It could be the expectations from their families to provide the basic necessities such as food, clothing, and shelter. And let's not forget the expectations of filing tax returns.

The fast-paced society we live in is all about being expeditious. Everything has to be done quickly and efficiently, and it is indoctrinated into us from a very early age. It may be school, where learning is thrust upon children via a uniform education system that does not normally take into account each child's learning abilities or difficulties. This also comes from the perils and pressures of performing well in standardized tests in order to be able to secure their future, and especially of ensuring prospects for higher education that could lead to a dream career. A person's life from adolescence to adulthood is spent in constant worry. Assignments, exams, projects, grades, reports—all of these continually hover over us like the Sword of Damocles.

There are several reasons why our stress levels are magnified as compared to the days of our ancestors. With the growing population, the era of competition at the turn of the 20th century prompted us all to get ahead of the others if we wanted to secure our future. Pursuing these goals became a rat race wherein we are never settling for less than the best. And in pursuit of these goals, we lose out on opportunities to destress and enrich our lives with healthier pursuits such as travel, exercise, hobbies, and recreation. Due to this, we become irritable, panicked, and even depressed.

WHY WE ARE STRESSED

The unparalleled pressure put upon us by modern society manifests itself in different ways and we are hardwired not to recognize it as problematic because this is how things are supposed to be. It could be a mammoth workload in order to achieve productivity gains, an obsession with getting ahead of the rest of the competition, and the never-ending search for perfection in everything we do. Because of this, we find ourselves with an unhealthy work-life balance and end up spending late nights at work, leaving our families neglected and a lot of cold dinners on the dining table. A lack of our personal presence not only creates an absence of your value in their lives, but also an absence of their positivity in ours.

As it happens, stress isn't only an externally-affecting condition. In fact, stress is an inherent biological reaction to all the events around us. Though there are several external situations that trigger it, it is important to remember that stress is actually your defense mechanism. It is necessary, but it should not be allowed to overwhelm you completely. In all creatures, including humans, stress is an evolutionary form of the "fight-or-flight" reflex which helps species survive. Even with the early humans who were hunters and gatherers, this reflex allowed them to overcome the odds.

Stress isn't just limited to upsetting experiences or events such as losing a job, not getting paid on time, tension in a relationship, divorce, and the death of a loved one. Stress can also occur in happy situations such as during a wedding, the birth of your first child, sending your kids to a new school, meeting a major prospective client, and even traveling to a new place. All these events affect us at a physical, psychological, and social level. The amount of stress that is triggered could either be considerable or otherwise. It could be a temporary state or could turn out to be recurring. Furthermore, our reactions to the sources of stress aren't the same as the next person, so it is crucial to recognize how your stress is triggered and how to face it.

These reactions occur normally as part of a fight-or-flight reflex in the case of a stressful event. According to evolutionary psychologists, this response helps us survive by analyzing a dangerous situation quickly. It tells your body that you are in trouble by increasing the levels of adrenaline almost immediately. This provides you with a considerable amount of energy and willpower to be able to choose the best course of action. This could either be to run away (flight) or face it (fight). The most common signs that your fight-or-flight reflex has activated includes an increased heart rate, shaking or trembling, pupil dilation, an increase in body temperature and blood pressure, clammy hands, pale or flushed skin, and most importantly, a sense of shock. Apart from these signs, you may also feel an interruption in the digestion process as well as some other important bodily functions.

The spike in your adrenaline also creates a sense of hyperawareness, which allows you to become more aware of your surroundings, particularly any movement in your peripheral vision and noises that are low in volume. It is almost as if you are in slow motion, like you may have seen in action movies. This is because the neurons in your brain are accelerating at a quicker pace in order to let you consider all the possibilities and variables for you to make your decision. The adrenal gland floods its hormones through you and there is an extra rush of blood to your muscles, particularly those that could aid you if you choose to run.

Once the stress-inducing event has been resolved, your body can take up to an hour to revert back to its normal state of homeostasis. However, this also leads to tiredness and exhaustion because of the exertion, not to mention a feeling of anxiety or apprehension as to whether the problem is actually gone or not. Furthermore, repeated or recurring fight-or-flight responses to stressful situations can cause hyperglycemia which may lead to hypertension or Type 2 diabetes.

Unfortunately, the fast-paced world we live in provides ample opportunities for people to get stressed. It could be preparing for a speech or presentation, loud or unexpected noises, meeting a potential new partner or going on a first date, seeing or being in a car accident, and so on. Even though most of these situations are not life-threatening, the fight-or-flight response kicks in every time there is a stressful incident. In situations where you do decide to fight and your body is required to exert itself physically, your adrenaline rush may cause you to perform feats of extraordinary strength, such as responding to a disaster and helping people who are trapped. Though you may not know it at the time, such exertion can lead to muscle tissue damage that will take a long time to heal.

SIGNS OF STRESS

Whenever we face a stressful situation, our body releases various hormones, such as adrenaline, as a response. We may also notice symptoms such as anxiety and distress. These can feel like a knot in your stomach, a lump in your throat, palpitations or a racing heartbeat. Though these are all short-term symptoms, prolonged and uncontrolled stress can actually cause damage to your overall health and well-being. You may face ailments including digestive disorders, irritability, agitation, sleep disorders, depression, muscular tension, burnout, isolation, problems in your relationships, lower performance at work, absenteeism, and a loss of self-esteem. This could ultimately lead to the development of critical diseases such as heart and vascular diseases, and cancer.

It's also important to remember that your nervous system cannot directly distinguish if the threats you face are emotional or physical. Your body is bound to react just as strongly no matter if you are in an argument with a friend or in a life-or-death situation. Because our stress mechanism is triggered so often these days, we may end up in a heightened state of stress so much that it becomes our normal resting state. This leads to serious health problems that cause disruptions to our immune, digestive, and reproductive systems. It may also increase the risk of heart attacks or strokes, and could also accelerate the aging process. Not to mention that the effects on your brain will cause you to be more anxious and depressed. You will constantly be doubting yourself. Such health problems also contribute to a lack of sleep, weight problems, eating disorders, and skin conditions.

Skin conditions such as acne are the most visible indicators of stress. Notice how often you touch your face whenever you are stressed, presumably with sweaty hands. Such frequent touching can easily spread bacteria across your face, resulting in acne. The hormonal shifts inside your body could also contribute to acne development. Stress is known to cause headaches. This is because your mind is thinking over everything related to the event that is causing the stress. Headaches, as well as tension in the neck, become quite frequent and chronic as we move about our lives without getting an adequate balance between work and home. They are further exacerbated due to lack of sleep or rest and dehydration, which are things we tend to ignore whenever we are stressed.

The constant exertion also leads to pains and aches across the body, such as in our joints, limbs, and back. Constant work on computers, laptops, and smartphones can lead to repetitive stress injuries that affect our hands, wrists, fingers, and neck. People on their feet at job sites often experience aches in their feet and lower limbs from constant movement and standing for long periods. Other factors such as poor posture, untended injuries, lack of proper nutrition, and nerve damage can contribute to these chronic pains.

Furthermore, you may also notice a spike in illnesses or allergies such as a runny nose, colds, sore throats, and fevers, which are all tell-tale signs of stress. Because it takes a toll on your immune system, you become more susceptible to infections. One study showed that adults with chronic stress showed a weaker immune response to flu vaccines, which suggests a compromised immune system. Another study showed a group of people categorized with high stress to be more susceptible to respiratory infections. Though more studies are required to sufficiently link stress to the wearing down of immune health, other factors such as poor diet or overexertion because of stress also contribute to a weakened immune system.

Loss of energy levels and chronic fatigue are also the most debilitating of the stress indicators, and certainly the most frustrating. How often have you found yourself in a high-stress situation where you are up against a deadline but simply no longer have the energy to complete the assignment? We become agitated with ourselves because our body can no longer cope with the demands of the task at hand and we keep pushing it, resulting in insomnia, digestive problems, and mental fatigue. Factors such as restlessness while trying to sleep, low blood sugar, and dehydration also cause a rapid depletion in energy.

High levels of stress also cause digestive issues such as diarrhea, constipation, stomach aches, bloating, irritable bowel syndrome (IBS), or inflammatory bowel disease (IBD). Aside from how stress can affect your digestion, it can also induce changes in your appetite which may cause you to either have no appetite at all or have a voracious one that will have you eating comfort food every moment you get. Even if you aren't hungry, you may end up overloading yourself with unhealthy food just as a distraction. Conversely, you may actually avoid eating when you need it the most, particularly when your energy reserves are depleting. Ultimately, that also affects your digestive system as well as losses or gains in weight.

If that doesn't say enough about how detrimental stress can be to you, consider what it can do to your sex drive. Whether you are a man or a woman, stress can actually hamper your libido and arousal, not to mention the levels of sexual satisfaction even if your partner is delivering completely. You probably won't be in the mood if all you are thinking about is the amount of work you have left at the office. Depression also affects your general interest in things. Both acute and chronic stress lead towards depression. Symptoms include apathy, disinterest, irritability, and so on. Environmental factors, family history, the type of crowd you associate with, and the kind of conversations and discussions you find yourself a part of can also contribute greatly towards depression, not to mention the effect of certain medications.

Increased heart rate is also a symptom of high stress levels as our fight-or-flight reaction elevates the heartbeat. Undergoing stressful tasks or having to deal with both personal and professional confrontations with high stakes results in the heart pumping more and more blood throughout your body; this means your heart rate is rapidly increasing. This is also because of high blood pressure, thyroid disease, certain heart conditions, and also the increased consumption of caffeinated or alcoholic beverages. You may start sweating more frequently and having increased body odor. People with existing conditions such as palmar hyperhidrosis, a condition where a person sweats excessively from their hands, face even more sweating because of stress.

THE ROLE OF CORTISOL

Despite how stress disrupts our regular life, it is usually exacerbated because of the buildup of cortisol in our brain. Cortisol is a naturally occurring hormone that has multiple functions, such as regulating blood sugar levels in the cells. It also contributes greatly to the function of the hippocampus, a part of the brain instrumental in storing and processing memories. Due to chronic stress, the body ends up making more cortisol than it can release, which can wear down the brain's functioning capabilities.

Stress has been observed to disrupt synapse regulation. This can cause a lack of sociability and dislike in social interactions. It can also kill brain cells and has a shrinking effect on the prefrontal cortex, which is the area of the brain that is responsible for learning and memory. As the prefrontal cortex shrinks, the size of the amygdala increases because of stress, making the brain even more agitated in stressful situations. This will ultimately lead you towards depression as well as poor coping abilities and physical illness. Stress can prove to be overwhelming if you have poor coping skills, which can cause a constant bad mood and decrease in productivity, not to mention trouble with your personal relationships.

REDUCING STRESS

The key here is to be able to properly manage your stress in order to avoid the harmful effects it can potentially cause. On a positive note, stress is actually useful if you need to improve or boost your concentration upon a task. In this case, it helps to increase your productivity and may enhance your creativity. Under stress, we find new and creative methods to work smart, not hard, which also leads to developing new skills such as time management, prioritization, delegation, and so on. First, keep in mind that everyone reacts differently to stress, so there isn't just one particular method to manage it. Therefore you need to learn how to gain control over it using a method that suits you so that you are able to manage it properly.

Let's start with recognizing what exactly triggers your stress. Once you identify those triggers, keep a sharp eye out for the symptoms we reviewed above and make note of which of those affect you the most. Then you should start discussing the cause of your stress (i.e., the problems themselves) with people who have your best interests at heart and whose judgment you can trust. This will help you a great deal as your stress automatically lessens once you unburden yourself with someone who will listen to you without judging or interrupting. If the need arises, you should also consult with a professional therapist to get a more informed opinion as well as learn about effective techniques to manage your stress.

It is also helpful to discuss the issues that are driving you up the wall, especially if they are work-related. Having a conversation with your co-workers, particularly your peers or immediate managers, can help you bring the issues out in the open. This will also provide you with an opportunity to get much-needed input from a different perspective. Because stress tends to hinder our perception of things, it never hurts to get a fresh set of eyes to look into the problem. Also, being in a leadership role puts a different kind of stress on you that requires ensuring that the task or project succeeds, in which case you might want to hold your cards close to your chest. However, by being trusting of your team's abilities, you should be able to easily delegate any tasks that you feel can be assigned. This helps take a lot of pressure off of you and also shows you to be a capable leader.

Different exercise techniques are known to release the tension that builds up due to stress and can go a long way to help you regain your sense of composure and clarity. It could be doing high-intensity exercise or taking a yoga class, going out for a pleasant walk in the park or even hitting a punching bag. You will feel the tension venting out every time you decide to take a moment and escape from the situation that is causing you stress. Your mind also plays a part, as letting things get to you also causes a lot of stress, particularly the things that are out of your control. Looking for alternatives or solutions should be your priority, rather than dwelling on what isn't working for you.

You should also look into how you can use your relaxation response. It actually isn't very hard to train your brain to relax in stressful situations, but it does require practice. The first thing you should do is take deep breaths and learn to control your breathing. Practice how you pace your breathing and you will be able to cool down whenever the symptoms and signs of stress start becoming obvious. Of course, that doesn't mean you need to dive head-first into stressful situations just so you can practice this. Breathing exercises can be practiced when you are calm. This will help you to regain your focus and clarity whenever you are actually in a stressful situation. You're training your brain to associate these breathing exercises with a sense of calm. This will make it easier to think back to a calmer and happier state when faced with a stressful situation.

Another very important, but relatively unknown stress response, is called "freeze and fawn," which is commonly associated with fight or flight. This is displayed by animals such as opossums that "play dead" whenever they sense danger from a predator. Sensing them in a freeze state, the predators will likely leave them alone as there is no sport in it for them. This is where the famous adage "playing possum" comes from. Opossums are incredibly well-skilled at making no movements whatsoever in the freeze state. The other response is fawn, which is an adrenal reaction to being pushed into a situation where you find it easier to give in. This is where the "yes man" mentality comes in and they decide that the person making the demand is correct and therefore it is what they should do. Because of the fawn state, we immediately say yes and accept our fate. This can happen when your manager asks you to stay late and you automatically agree even if you really don't want to or have other plans.

So whether you fall under the category of fight, flight, freeze, or fawn, it is likely that you are faced with stressful situations in your life, both at home and at work. It is also likely that you may be dealing negatively with these situations, which is why it is recommended to find a healthier or safer environment that will keep you away from stressful situations. Spending time with your family or even taking time for yourself to engage in hobbies helps a lot with de-stressing. Creative hobbies such as art, writing, crafting, working on do-it-yourself projects, and so on prove to be therapeutic, as do doing chores around the house and organizing.

And here's something you may not have considered: Taking the time to properly poop. Oh yes, we are definitely going there. As we have seen before, research is unearthing the link between stress and constipation. Stress can trigger or exacerbate gastrointestinal symptoms such as stomach pain, nausea, irregular bowel movements, and constipation. Researchers have observed that the stress hormone could contribute to constipation as some of the common causes include dehydration, poor diet, insufficient fiber intake, and a lack of physical activity. When you find yourself in a stressful situation, a hormone called epinephrine is released from your adrenal glands, which plays a role in your fight-or-flight response. This hormone causes the body to divert blood flow to the vital organs from the intestines, which results in a slowdown in your intestinal movements.

Along with epinephrine, the body also releases corticotropin-releasing factor (CRF) in the bowels, which can further slow down intestinal movements and even cause the intestines to become inflamed. Additionally, stress can cause an increase in intestinal permeability which allows inflammatory compounds to enter the intestines. This results in a feeling of abdominal fullness. The result: constipation.

Psychological stress leads to physical symptoms such as constipation. It is called a somatic symptom and may be observed if you have less than three bowel movements per week, or if they are difficult or painful. It may even feel like you are not able to empty your bowels. This results in dry or lumpy stool. Furthermore, stress is likely to cause you to eat an unhealthy diet as well as forgo sleep or exercise. Worse still, you may even forget to stay hydrated. All of these can contribute to constipation.

In order to treat stress-related constipation, you should seriously consider improving your diet by eating a lot of fiber and drinking plenty of fluids. Avoiding items high in sugar and fat, as well as cigarettes and alcohol, reduces the chances of constipation and stress. Along with that, keep yourself physically active through exercise; this way, you will be able to make sure your intestinal movements continue.

And as we've seen earlier, such measures can also greatly help your mental health in order to manage your stress levels.

2

THE IMPACTS OF FOOD ON YOUR BODY

"Let food be thy medicine and medicine be thy food."

— HIPPOCRATES

How often do you consider the importance of food? How many times have you been out with friends at a restaurant or enjoying takeout at your place as you watch a basketball game on TV and thought about what you were eating? Aside from taking a few food snaps for your social media account, how much importance do you actually place on your food? Do you know what's in it? Do you know where the ingredients came from? Do you even think about what those ingredients are doing to your body or how they are impacting both your physical as well as mental health?

The food you eat every day has a major impact on all aspects of your health. Whether it is physical, mental, or even emotional, the ingredients within these foods affect us with various chemical reactions and changes that trigger certain responses within us at a base level. The way food is provided to us in modern times is mostly packaged and loaded with preservatives from various corporate enterprises. The ingredients in most foods now make us sluggish, lethargic, unmotivated, depressed, and even sick. Despite this, we take very little interest in what we are consuming and simply purchase whatever suits our tastes. Moreover, most doctors have only rudimentary knowledge about food and are more likely to prescribe medications or supplements rather than suggesting healthy food.

In the last decade, however, there has been a seismic shift towards eating healthy and organic food, particularly food that hasn't been mass-manufactured or packaged. These nutritious foods are becoming more widely available in supermarkets. Moreover, political activism against health issues stemming from overeating, high cholesterol, and obesity has started to pick up steam in powerful corridors, and there is a renewed interest in the science of functional foods.

THE ROLE OF BIG PHARMA

Despite the amount of research that goes into food development, as well as the amount of quality checks involved with approving and assigning food certifications, the Western world has the highest rate of illnesses across a broad range. This includes high cholesterol, high blood pressure, high blood sugar, obesity, diabetes, heartburn, gastroesophageal and reflux disease, most of which comes from overconsumption of junk food. Not only that, the population also suffers from physical ailments such as backaches, joint pain, poor blood circulation, and also sleep apnea. This is due to the extra weight we gain from eating junk food that ends up as unhealthy fat in our body.

Lack of proper nutrition also creates deficiencies within our bodies which lead to other types of illnesses or medical conditions. These include asthma, seasonal allergies, irritable bowel syndrome, dry eye, fibromyalgia, insomnia, migraines, chronic fatigue, restless legs, osteopenia, perimenopause, lactose intolerance, and even erectile dysfunction. Moreover, we can also face challenges with our mental health, such as obsessive-compulsive disorders, spectrum disorders, excessive daytime sleepiness, social anxiety, depression, bipolar disorder, attention deficit hyperactivity disorder, and so on.

But why do we have such malnutrition among the population? The widespread availability of fast food everywhere has made it the go-to meal in any situation. This is the case in both major cities and smaller towns. Not only are they common restaurants, now fast food chains are in malls, theaters, food courts, office parks, and even hospitals of all places. Moreover, the variety of serving sizes in the meals such as super-sizing, upsizing, free refills, combo meals, and all-you-can-eat buffets tempt people with several options that are easily affordable. Upgrades are made even more convincing by the advertisements for the savings patrons would make with the bigger deals. The concept of portion control and restraint is dying out as many people no longer have family meals where everyone eats the same thing. Now, food is instantly ordered and delivered at any hour of the day, and can be easily microwaved to be consumed whenever we feel like it.

No matter what the disease or deficiency that we may be facing, pharmaceutical companies are always at hand with a solution. If the marketing is to be believed, we will continue to need these medicinal solutions for the rest of our lives. There is always a pill available that can treat our obesity or help us control our blood sugar or anything else that ails us. You may have noticed press releases and TV ads that claim to raise awareness about an under-recognized disease that could jeopardize your health. The ads point out the various symptoms and risks. Listening to these may make you feel as if you are already suffering from more than one of these symptoms. This leads you to self-diagnose yourself and even check online to find out if you are actually are suffering from the disease. You may even end up at an official website where you are asked to take a quiz just to confirm your suspicions. And before you know it, you have found yourself hooked on a drug regimen that you may not have even needed.

What has become apparent is that diseases and deficiencies that barely got the time of day not long ago are now being marketed en masse for the sole purpose of creating the need for new pharmaceutical products. According to noted cardiologist and author Dr. Aseem Malhotra, there needs to be a change in European health policy regarding lifestyle medicine. Being a leading figure against sugar and widespread medicine usage, Dr. Malhotra believes that prescribed medications do a lot more harm than good as people are taking pills they do not really need. This in turn causes a detrimental effect on people's lives, making prescribed medicines the third biggest killer after heart disease and cancer, Dr. Malhotra says.

As part of a campaign against excess sugar and medicine usage in Britain, Dr. Malhotra has shed light on the coordinated efforts of the food and beverage industry as well as the pharmaceutical industries to influence government policy for their benefit. This involves getting doctors to prescribe medications that may not even be necessary in lieu of basic lifestyle changes. Furthermore, such actions may even involve potentially harmful treatments. According to statistics, more than half of all adults in the United Kingdom are taking at least one prescription medication. Out of this number, 50% of the people over the age of 70 are taking at least three medications. The campaign cites that unscrupulous lobbying practices by pharmaceutical concerns have been creating major conflicts of interests at the highest level. These activities have put evidence-based medicine on the back burner and focused solely on profits rather than public health and safety.

THE GUT-BRAIN AXIS

The amount of foods with processed sugar, meat, dairy, and refined grains that are readily available in supermarkets and restaurants do a great deal of damage to both your physical and mental health. Consuming such food items on a regular basis has been known to cause conditions such as gut dysbiosis, which may ultimately cause depression. As we saw in the previous chapter, our body redirects a tremendous amount of energy and resources to the muscles and the brain in response to a stressful event, along with releasing cortisol. All of these factors wreak havoc on the gut microbiome. Similarly, your mood can be affected because of stress and anxiety when your gut microbiome is imbalanced (i.e., dysbiosis).

Your stress resilience is actually improved if your gut microbiome is balanced. If imbalanced, there is a direct impact on your mental health due to a major part of your autonomic nervous system called the vagus nerve, which connects your gut and your brain. This nerve is responsible for sending messages to and from your brain and colon; it is essential for your mental health. Any undue stress on the connection between your brain and gut can lead towards illnesses that affect your brain, as well as irritable bowel syndrome (IBS).

The vagus nerve aids digestion in numerous ways. It allows organisms to move independently using metabolic energy, otherwise known as motility. This helps food to move through the digestive tract with ease. Furthermore, the vagus nerve stimulates the release of digestive enzymes which are necessary for proper digestion and also communicates your body's appetite to the brain. It also detects gut bacteria that break down the food, such as dietary fiber, and transforms it into metabolites. Metabolites such as short-chain fatty acids (SCFAs) are also detected by the nerve, which in turn informs the brain to allow proper digestive regulation.

Simply put, your brain and your gut are in constant communication through the vagus nerve which helps to regulate both your digestion and your moods. If stress manages to impair this nerve, it becomes unable to react to inflammation. This occurs because your gut microbiome is not balanced which results in dysbiosis. Inflammation is caused due to microbes proliferating. Due to this, your digestion is affected and your gut and gut bacteria also come under attack. Not only that, you automatically experience unhappiness and depression due to the inflammation. Depression can also compound your inflammation.

Therefore, by controlling inflammation, you can actually help to improve your anxiety levels as well as stabilize your mood. But what does that have to do with the food that you are buying? In order to balance your gut microbiome, it is necessary to increase the abundance of diverse microbes that will actually help to reduce inflammation. A good source of such helpful bacteria is following a natural, plant-based diet. Having a steady course of fruits, vegetables, nuts, seeds, whole grains, legumes, and so on not only keeps your gut happy, but also improves the link between your gut and your brain, resulting in better mental health.

Another source of beneficial bacteria are probiotics that provide numerous health benefits, especially to your mental health. Though they naturally reside in the gut, they may also be obtained from fermented foods such as yogurt and kefir, as well as other supplements. A field called psychobiotics explores the link between probiotics and mental health, and research has shown that probiotics such as Lactobacillus improve stress resilience as well as reduce anxiety. Other probiotics such as Bifidobacterium and Lactococcus help to alleviate the symptoms of depression and support your physical health. The reason why probiotics are good for overall health is that they keep the gut ecosystem balanced, preventing gut dysbiosis.

In the same vein, you would also want to nourish your growing probiotic bacteria in order to get all the health benefits. Prebiotics are found in foods such as onions, berries, apples, seeds, garlic, legumes, potatoes, cocoa, mushrooms, green bananas, barley, corn, and many more. The gut bacteria is nourished by prebiotic fibers, polyphenols, and resistant starches, and are transformed into SCFAs and vitamins that benefit your health.

Ultimately, a well-balanced gut ecosystem helps to protect your mental health because of the helpful bacteria in your gut. By nourishing them sufficiently, the gut produces chemicals such as serotonin that regulate your mood, anxiety levels, and happiness levels.

THE ROLE OF NUTRITION

So why do people not realize that a cheeseburger is not really nourishing the body? Why do they feel that way too many french fries won't make them sick?

The better question here is: How often do people actually consider which foods are actually good for their health. With the speed at which life moves these days, we hardly ever consider the ingredients in the food we are eating and, chances are, we finish eating before the thought can even cross our mind. Moreover, there is a lack of general education and awareness about healthy food in schools. There is even a lack of public service announcements.

In a study called the "2020 State of Healthy Eating in America" released by Del Monte Foods, one in three Americans admit that they did not learn about nutrition at any level of their education. Moreover, they have never considered or even thought about what foods would be best for their health, as they believe that anything available in the market should be good enough. 70% of Americans believe that eating a healthy diet enables them to be the best version of themselves, while 32% of the younger generation feel a great deal of anxiety and social pressure over what they eat.

As the 21st century progresses, it is clear that Americans are of different minds when it comes to food and nutrition, particularly what constitutes as healthy for them. Research shows that 69% of Americans feel that they need to make sacrifices to allow for healthy eating. They believe that this means missing out on the fun of fast food and eating out, while 30% believe that the only way they could afford healthy food would be to cut down on visiting restaurants. Many think that healthy eating is actually very expensive. That said, one in five Americans finds it difficult to cancel their streaming service subscriptions in order to be able to afford healthy food.

On the other hand, the study also reveals that 78% of Americans think that fresh food is healthy, but 13% also believe that packaged food is. Meanwhile, 58% of Americans state that they are not able to properly store fresh food in their home. Not only that, one in three people find it to be a waste of money as improper storage leads to it spoiling quickly. This is even after the Produce for Better Health Foundation recommended at least five servings of fruits and vegetables daily. These include fresh, frozen, canned, or dried. Juice is also recommended. The nutritional benefits offered here are generally consistent and have proven to improve health and the quality of diet.

Companies such as Del Monte that primarily focus on plant-based foods feel that it is necessary to impart knowledge and facts about healthy eating starting from elementary school and later at the middle-school level throughout the country. This way, every new generation would be able to make conscious decisions about their health choices and choose options that encourage better mental and physical well-being.

Aside from the availability of healthy and fresh food in the market, the variable individual diet requirements based on one's health and existing medical conditions make a uniform diet a challenging prospect. The sheer volume of customized diet plans out there creates even more confusion for people who are already concerned about how to go about having a healthy lifestyle. Nevertheless, there are some universal precautions people can take and food that people can avoid in order to grasp the fundamentals of nutrition.

For instance, meat bought at supermarkets is very likely to be filled with growth hormones that are part-and-parcel of the meat production industry. Livestock being raised by the meat industry is heavily regulated by growth hormones in order to control aspects such as growth, feeding requirements, milk production, and also the quantity and quality of fat and muscle. These practices have become so widespread that it is actually cheaper to raise livestock on growth hormones rather than natural nutrition. This also increases the profit of the meat itself.

However, these hormones may also include exogenous sex hormones that are actually carcinogenic to humans. For example, any milk obtained from cows that have received exogenous hormones cannot be sold commercially. Therefore, the use of such hormones in food products such as meat and dairy is either strictly controlled in most cases, or completely prohibited in some. Other growth hormones found in meat could affect prepubescent children who are not producing growth hormones yet themselves. A study has found that by ingesting these growth hormones through meat or dairy products, children may enter puberty much earlier than usual.

While several studies have shown that the existence of hormones in human and animal milk is vital for growth and immunity in infants, further evidence over time suggests that hormones in dairy may have a detrimental impact on human health. This could be the result of some estrogens and insulin-like growth factor 1 that may be responsible for breast, prostate, and endometrial tumors. Therefore, recent studies show that there are some hormones in milk that act as biomarkers for diseases.

And let's not forget the biggest repeat offender: gluten. It could be a sugary, fried doughnut or an organic 12-grain loaf of bread—gluten is everywhere and affects your gut the same way no matter what food it is in. And it is not good, as gluten can do a lot of damage to your intestine. By the time your meal reaches the intestines, an enzyme is produced in your intestinal wall that breaks down gluten into its protein building blocks, gliadin and glutenin. This enzyme is called tissue transglutaminase (tTG). It has other responsibilities, such as holding the microvilli in our gut together, and these microvilli perform the crucial task of absorbing nutrients from the intestine walls.

The problem arises in people who are sensitive to gluten. The proteins travel through your digestive system and the gut-associated lymphoid tissue (GALT) checks the proteins for any harmful substances. While the proteins are absorbed in people who are not gluten-sensitive, this is not the case if there is gluten sensitivity. This is when the GALT marks gliadin as a harmful substance and therefore produces antibodies to attack it. For people who have celiac disease, the antibodies also attack the tTG along with the gliadin, and, considering its crucial role, this attack could leave your microvilli devastated.

Because your microvilli can no longer absorb the nutrients, the intestinal walls become leaky which creates further digestive issues such as bloating, constipation, diarrhea, weight loss, and fat malabsorption. Furthermore, it can also cause malnutrition including iron deficiency, anemia, low vitamin D, and even osteoporosis. Other hazards of having a leaky gut include releasing of toxins, microbes, antibodies, and undigested food particles from your intestines into your bloodstream. Remember, these are the same antibodies that attack the gliadin and tTG in the first place. What's more, these antibodies don't just mistake tTG for gliadin but also other organs and systems such as the skin, thyroid, and brain.

The best way to find out if you are sensitive to gluten is to go without. By eliminating it completely from your diet for at least 30 days, you can then check your gluten sensitivity by reintroducing it. If you feel worse, then it is a clear indication that you are sensitive regardless of a negative test result.

Know Your Whole Grains

A sure-fire way to make your diet healthier is by eating more whole grains. These contain many beneficial nutrients and provide a powerful variety of protein, fiber, B vitamins, and antioxidants, not to mention trace minerals such as iron, zinc, copper, and magnesium. Whole-grain diets provide a variety of benefits such as reducing the risks of heart disease, Type 2 diabetes, obesity, and certain kinds of cancer. They are also known to help with bowel health as fiber helps maintain regular bowel movements and invigorates the growth of healthy bacteria in the colon.

However, it is surprising to know that over 40% of Americans do not eat any whole grains at all. The average American eats less than one serving on a daily basis, and this also includes young adults. Most people are of the opinion that whole grains are difficult to add to their daily diets, and also that they don't actually taste good. Furthermore, they get rather confused when it comes to picking out foods that are whole-grain. Anytime they are at a supermarket, they get caught up in the packaging of different products such as bread, cereal, or even healthy snacks. Almost all of them claim to promote whole-grain goodness, but that is not entirely true. The terms vary such as multigrain, cracked wheat, organic, 100% wheat, bran, pumpernickel, and stone-ground. And, while all of them sound like they are brimming with the benefits of grain, none of these labels actually confirm that they are whole-grain.

Each whole grain comprises the bran, germ, and endosperm that are all edible parts. It can either be used intact or recombined, as long as all the components are naturally proportionate. A good idea is to keep a list handy with you on your next trip to the supermarket, and select grains such as whole-grain corn, whole oats, brown rice, whole rye, whole-grain barley, wild rice, buckwheat, triticale, bulgur, millet, quinoa, sorghum, 100% whole wheat flour, and, an all-time favorite, popcorn.

One thing to be mindful of is that whenever you buy processed wheat products, such as loaves of bread, they have mostly been stripped of the outer layer of bran from the whole kernel of wheat. Once the refined wheat flour is obtained, molasses is added to color it brown and they are then packaged as "100% wheat" bread. That does not make it whole-grain, which is why it is important to check the packaging labels, particularly the words that come after "whole." The ingredients list should have whole grain as the first ingredient with a clear indication that it has more whole grain by weight than the rest of the ingredients. According to the 2010 USDA Dietary Guidelines, whole grains should make up half of your grain intake, though the amount may vary based on individual parameters such as age, gender, and physical activity level.

Another lesser known fact is that whole grains don't have to be brown, nor do they have to be multigrain or only in adult cereals. Many processed foods do contain whole grains as there has been an increase in whole-grain options for foods like cereals and pastas. A lot of restaurants offer brown rice as well as other whole-grain options, and some processed foods are being reformulated with lighter whole wheat and new processing techniques to eliminate the "grainy" taste that most people are put off by. If nothing else, people can use these white whole-grain options to get a feel for it before transitioning into eating more whole grains.

This is especially helpful if your kids are pretty fond of sliced white bread.

Not all whole grains are brimming with fiber. Whole wheat contains the highest amount of fiber, brown rice contains the least. The majority of whole-grain sources contain about one to four grams of fiber per serving which is comparable to the quantity found in fruit and vegetables. This makes whole grains a good source of fiber for most people. They are far more beneficial nutritionally than fiber supplements. Nevertheless, fiber supplements could be used if you aren't getting the required amount of fiber daily. The required amount is 25 grams per day for women and 38 grams per day for men.

Because whole grains taste and feel different, it does take a bit of time to adjust to eating them without feeling put off. Whole-grain breads, cereals, crackers, and bagels can help you easily acclimatize to the taste. You can make simple sandwiches using whole-grain breads like whole meal, wheat germ, multigram, granary, seeded, or mixed-grain. There are also whole-wheat pita wraps that offer more variety and taste. Grain cereals make a great breakfast as long as the sugar quantity is kept to a minimum. As for something fun, low-fat, air-popped popcorn could be the perfect snack, so long as it isn't pre-popped or covered with salt, butter, cheese, or other unhealthy toppings.

On the subject of snacks, other options could include rye crackers, whole-grain rice cakes, and oatcakes. Check the labels and ingredients thoroughly to make sure they are not too high in sodium, fats, and calories. It's also a good idea to bake your cakes, pastries, and pies with whole grains added to them. Blending half whole-meal flour with all-purpose flour helps you boost the content of whole grains in your baked goods. You can also replace one-third of your flour with whole-grain oats and buy brown rice as well as whole-wheat or blended pasta. There are also some lesser known whole grains such as barley, brown rice, millet, quinoa, or sorghum that can be used in risottos, whole-grain salads, pilafs, and so on. And if you have kids, it helps to get them started on whole grains early so that they get used to the flavor. You can try out buns made out of whole grains the next time you're making burgers, or even use whole-wheat pitas as a pizza base.

3

HONOR THE SUN GODDESS

I t's a bright, sunny day. At least, that's what everyone says. But have you ever stopped to wonder why they say that? What exactly does the sun do that makes people look upbeat and excited about the possibilities that the day holds? Back in grade school, you must have learned about how the sun works miracles for plant growth. You may have even noticed how plants in your garden would always spurt out and point in the direction of the sunlight. The sun enriches all life on Earth, including humans. It affects growth and strength, and also affects your emotional state in ways you may not even realize. Just standing outside in the sunlight makes you feel good and warm on the inside, even if it's a windy or chilly day.

Think about it. How often do you find yourself down in the dumps on a rainy or snowy day when there isn't much daylight? In those situations, the world appears to be quite gray and so does your outlook. Or even when you are indoors at work, cooped up in your monochrome office space and taking on stress upon stress, you long for a quick moment just to step outside the building. And what happens when you do? You feel instantly energized and happy, not to mention motivated enough to go back and overcome the challenges that had been weighing you down. Venturing out to the beach and lying in the sun, or going to a particularly sunny travel destination for your vacation feels like such a relief, and you returned recharged.

You might have some idea of how sunlight accomplishes this by generating a healthy amount of vitamin D for all living creatures. In fact, 90% of all vitamin D comes to us directly from the sun, while the rest of it comes from food sources or supplements. It has amazing health benefits. It helps to absorb calcium in our bodies, thereby leading to healthy bone growth. It also helps to strengthen your immune system and promotes good oral health.

But did you know that vitamin D actually contributes a great deal to our mental health as well? Aside from all the physical and medical health benefits, vitamin D keeps you in an upbeat mood and helps to ensure a state of happiness. This way, it is instrumental in fighting off depression naturally, particularly seasonal depression that occurs during the cooler seasons.

As adults, we tend not to express our happiness as readily as we used to when we were children. You may also see seasonal shifts in your mood and feel as if you are gloomier in winter than you are in the summertime. Because there are more hours of sunlight in the summer, you tend to get enough exposure to it that it helps lift your mood and you feel upbeat, even though you may be going through inner turmoil. You may also notice that as the sun sets, you get a feeling that this high appears to be coming to an end. And it becomes apparent even more when you are out in the winter season. Therefore, the importance of how much vitamin D affects our health and happiness should not be underestimated.

As if that weren't enough, vitamin D also acts as a natural appetite suppressant. This is ideal if you are looking to lose weight. Sitting in the sun for a little bit helps to alleviate or minimize your hunger pangs. Lack of exposure to sunlight can explain why you may be facing difficulties losing weight. Vitamin D helps in detoxifying the body by regulating your hormones and lowering fat storage levels. It also controls the level of serotonin in your body which affects your mood, your sleep regulation, and so on. This makes having healthy levels of vitamin D essential to feel more motivated, eat well, and have a great quality of life.

More often than not, you may be experiencing a short term depression that may actually be seasonal because of a lack of vitamin D. During such periods, your serotonin activity decreases; this puts you in a sad and gloomy state for most of the time. Nevertheless, that doesn't mean you need to immediately think about taking prescription medication to overcome the depression, as the answer may be as simple as stepping out into the daylight. However, the winter months may not offer a lot of sunlight, so it may be best to take a supplement.

Remember that vitamin D is a fat-soluble vitamin, so it is a good idea to speak to your doctor beforehand. You may be required to take a blood test to see if your vitamin D levels are indeed low. The reason is that the levels of vitamin D in supplements could prove to be toxic if they are too high for you. It is recommended that you learn what levels of vitamin D in your supplements are safe and right for you. Vitamin D supplements also need to be taken with a meal containing fat so that your body absorbs it properly.

THE IMPORTANCE OF VITAMIN D

Going out, exploring, being active, and a host of outdoor activities can help you enrich your vitamin D levels, which plays a direct role in boosting your energy levels. In turn, that gets you ready to become more active and the cycle continues. There is a direct correlation between vitamin D and staying physically active. These two factors combined will work together to give you the best results. Starting off your day with an early morning jog or a walk in the park, the rays of the sun will help you feel energized both physically as well as mentally. You will find you have a better grip over your feelings and a reduction in your depression and anxiety. Furthermore, exercises under the sun, especially in the morning, will lessen the time you need to recover from your workout.

You will also find your energy levels improving whenever you come home from work and decide to take a stroll in the park before the sun sets. This can also provide some much-needed bonding time with your children or even some time to yourself. You can perform mental exercises such as breathing exercises or meditation. If you are actively making space in your schedule, you can even perform high-intensity workouts, or interval training, where you work out with short bursts of energy followed by short periods of rest and then starting over again. These workouts provide better chances to reduce fat, build muscle, and improve endurance; they are further amplified by exposure to vitamin D.

One of the biggest disadvantages of living a sedentary lifestyle is the lack of exposure to adequate sunlight. If you are the kind of person who works a 9-to-5 job, you may simply be sitting in your car every morning fighting through traffic and then clocking in at your office building. More than likely you are in an air-conditioned environment in your car as well, simply to beat off the heat. And if that is the case, you may be complaining of terrible aches and pains in your body, particularly as you grow older. It could be in your joints, ankles, feet, legs, arms, and mostly your back and neck; these are more common because your body applies more pressure to your lower half while sitting down.

The reasons for this may vary. Perhaps you remain seated for long periods before you take your lunch break. Ideally, you should stand up and stretch out, maybe take a short stroll around the floor and then get back to work to keep yourself physically active. Alternatively, you could also use your coffee breaks to step outside the building or go out on the balcony just to get some fresh air and, of course, plenty of sunlight.

Having regulated levels of vitamin D as we grow older is important because it helps our intestines absorb calcium. This will also prevent our kidneys from excreting calcium.

Not getting enough of the sunshine vitamin may also lead to osteomalacia or osteoporosis, both of which could have severe consequences for your bone density and also cause muscular weakness. While osteomalacia is a softening of the bones, osteoporosis causes the bones to become brittle and porous hence the name literally meaning "porous bone." Similarly, it can also cause rickets in children, which is also a softening of bones in children.

Vitamin D also helps to reduce inflammation as well as regulate immune function and glucose metabolism. Furthermore, some studies have shown a reduction in risks of cancer and cardiovascular disease, though the results have been mixed.

The Journal of Nutrition and the The Journal of the American Osteopathic Association have both published studies that highlighted how people living in northern latitudes were found to have lower levels of vitamin D. This could include half of the United States, and the upper half of the northern hemisphere which get less sunlight exposure than other areas. Every moment people living in those regions spend out in the sun is precious. Another very important factor is age, as vitamin D cannot be as efficiently synthesized as our skin gets older and flaccid. With age, we see obvious signs of vitamin D deficiency such as aching bones, pain in muscles and joints, weakness, fatigues, and drowsiness. Vitamin D deficiency has also been traced among people with a body mass index (BMI) of 30 or higher. In such a situation, it is recommended to enter a manageable weight loss and diet plan and also increase vitamin D intake.

Realizing how important vitamin D is one thing, but we also need to understand just how important it is to make the most of the sunlight we get. During summertime, make sure you head outdoors as much as possible while the sun is shining. That is doubly important in winter, particularly on days that aren't cloudy. Keep checking your weather forecast apps to see what the best times are to soak in as much sunlight as you can. Foods such as salmon, mushrooms, and egg yolks contain natural vitamin D, and it can be found in fortified foods as well. Vitamin D is also available in dietary supplements which can be synthesized by the body whenever we step out into the sun.

Keep in mind that staying out of the sun or using too much sunblock can actually lead to a deficiency in vitamin D. Nevertheless, you should manage your exposure to the sun depending on the time of day, the climate, and the weather conditions in your region, and the time of year. Most people require anywhere from fifteen minutes to three hours of exposure to sunlight on a daily basis to get a sufficient dose of vitamin D. The amount of sun exposure you need will depend on your climate, the time of day, and the time of year.

People with lighter skin tend to absorb vitamin D more quickly. People with darker skin tones have greater quantities of melanin in their skin which gives them natural skin protection, but reduces the production of vitamin D in the skin. In fact, people with darker skin tones require at least three to five times more exposure to sunlight to get the required amount of vitamin D. However, supplementing your diet with foods rich in vitamin D as mentioned above could help to increase vitamin D levels.

If you follow all these steps, you will notice a natural uplift in your mood and overall happiness.

SHINING OUT DEPRESSION

A great deal of public interest is being shown in using vitamin D as a potential treatment for mental conditions such as depression and anxiety. These disorders can both be incredibly debilitating and detrimental to leading a normal and happy life. Though some research has shown that people with depression have been found with lower levels of vitamin D as opposed to people without depression, there is no clear conclusion that the vitamin can completely cure depression, certainly not one that has been found in a large-scale study.

Because there are various causes and symptoms of depression, there isn't exactly a single treatment that can alleviate the condition completely. Whether it is medications, vitamins, or other treatments, depression requires several different approaches which provide mixed results. While vitamin D is linked to treating depression, it does not exactly curb the symptoms of depression considering the increasing serum levels of the substance. Young people, the elderly, and those with chronic illnesses are all more susceptible to depression and vitamin D deficiency. Depression may lead to a vitamin D deficiency; this is particularly the case for those with tendencies of social withdrawal and who are lacking in self-care.

An increase in social interaction and a better diet can improve the symptoms of depression and levels of vitamin D, if for no other reason than to be out and about. Because of social withdrawal and isolation, not to mention loss in appetite, people suffering from depression may not go outdoors to restaurants or meet with people and therefore may not get the right amount of vitamin D. They may want to remain cooped up indoors and may even prefer staying in bed rather than coming out of their room. Symptoms of depression and vitamin deficiencies may worsen due to isolation and staying inside for extended periods. They may also not be practicing proper self-care which includes eating a proper and balanced diet. Ultimately, eating unhealthy food may inadvertently keep them from having any food fortified with vitamin D or other benefits.

Depression itself is a medical condition that has a negative effect on an individual's feelings, thoughts, and behaviors. But, it is actually a treatable disorder. Major depressive disorder can be mild, moderate, or severe in its intensity and the symptoms vary. The most noticeable symptoms include loss of appetite, excessive weight loss or gain, too little or too much sleep, lethargy, disruption in tasks, and poor concentration. There are also symptoms on a mental level such as isolation, anxiety, loss of interest in activities that were once enjoyable, overwhelming feelings of sadness, hopelessness, and helplessness, loss of sexual interest, and even contemplating suicidal thoughts or self-harm.

According to the American Psychiatric Association, depression affects an estimated one in fifteen adults at a rate of 6.7% in any given year. Furthermore, at least one in six people, or 16.6%, will experience some kind of depression in their lifetimes. Depression typically occurs during pre-teen and teen years, and can also manifest itself in early adulthood. It may also run in families as people with close relatives facing depression run a greater risk of developing depression themselves. Whether it is parents, siblings, or children, taking care of such relatives with depression often puts one under immense psychological strain. There are also genetic factors and similarities in biochemistry that can cause depression.

Other factors such as low self-esteem, self-doubt, or pessimism can also contribute greatly to depressive tendencies, as well as environmental factors such as punishment, neglect, or even physical abuse. Studies also show that women tend to develop depression more than men do, particularly due to hormonal changes related to pregnancy, menstruation, and also menopause. Statistics show that one in eight women, or 12.5%, are likely to experience depression at some point in their life.

Though a vitamin D deficiency can be easily determined by a blood test, the same cannot be said for depression. This requires an appointment with a doctor who will ask you questions about your symptoms and experiences to determine if you have a depressive disorder. Much like the symptoms, the steps you can take to alleviate depression also vary and can include joining a support group, reaching out to friends, family, and loved ones, exercising regularly, managing your sleep schedule, and talking with a licensed counselor. Support groups are a logical first step as they comprise people undergoing similar situations and symptoms. They can be attended in person, on the phone, or online, and are typically available in community centers.

The best therapy for the isolatory symptoms of depression could be reaching out to your loved ones, including your friends, family, partners, and so on. This would involve opening up about your feelings that are putting you in a depressive state. Not only that, but this depressive state could actually be caused by someone in your circle, so it is important to bring all of this out in the open so that you can all come together to help you come out of the present state. It is also important to make them understand what will not work so that they are aware of if and when their words or actions do not help your treatment. Exercising regularly helps by releasing chemicals such as endorphins which help our brain feel good. It can also reduce chemicals in the immune system that exacerbate the symptoms of depression, plus you also get to go out and get some fresh air and plenty of sunlight.

Similarly, getting good quality sleep on a regular schedule can help you cope with the symptoms of insomnia and hypersomnia, as well as other sleep issues that are linked to depression. There are simple steps you can follow, such as setting alarms and reminders for sleep and wake times on your phone, keeping a journal to log the duration and quality of your sleep every night so that you can track your progress, and listening to relaxation sounds such as nature sounds, hypnotic rhythms, and binaural beats.

LET THERE BE LIGHT

As we reviewed earlier, populations in the northern regions have a more complicated relationship with the sun. They tend to be affected more by depression because of the long and dark winter days with less daylight. In Scandinavian countries, such as Norway, the winter blues leave an impression on people who suffer from seasonal affective disorder (SAD), making winters literally depressing. This is an annually occurring condition that takes place at the same time each year and is regarded as a type of depression or bipolar disorder.

It even affects healthy people who do not show any signs of depression throughout the rest of the year, but they experience a dullness in mood and energy when fall begins and it continues through the winter. Regional historians often describe seasonal peaks of happiness and sadness going as far back as the sixth century, and it is always attributed to the increased daylight in the summer and the dramatic decrease of it in the winter, respectively.

The prevailing theory is that our circadian rhythms fall out of sync with the time of day because of shortened days during the winter season. Known as the phase-shift hypothesis, this leads to a delay in the release of melatonin in our body, which normally rises in response to darkness. With higher melatonin levels, we begin to feel sleepy until the bright light of the morning actually suppresses it. Due to the shorter hours of daylight in the winter, our levels of melatonin do not fall until later and our body begins feeling sleepy again or stays sleepy even when the alarm rings in the morning. Such a hormonal imbalance could have other unhealthy effects such as tiredness and depression.

4

THE IMPORTANCE OF SLEEP

"Are the children all in bed, for now it's eight o'clock?"

— *WEE WILLIE WINKIE* BY
WILLIAM MILLER

Think about your life when the sun sets. For many people that means coming home, maybe taking a shower, changing into new clothes, and starting an entirely new life. If they're highly sociable, they head out on the town and meet with friends over drinks and dinner. Maybe they'll check out the local bars to meet new people, head out on a date including dinner and a movie. Some might just stay at home and read a book or watch Netflix through the night.

For others, the nights are when they get to work, whether it is working from home or heading out to a graveyard shift. There may even be a second job late at night for supplementary income. Some may also do volunteer work at soup kitchens or other charities, or even enroll themselves in a skills course at night to enhance their knowledge and abilities for a prosperous career. So much can be accomplished in the night, after all, what else would you rather be doing? Sleeping?

Making use of the hours after the sun sets to be out and about doing all sorts of things as mentioned above requires a great deal of energy, particularly if you have already had a long day at work. And while you may be able to power through the hours after dark to accomplish your goals or maintain a steady social life, you are doing yourself an injustice by missing out on crucial sleep time that your body and mind so desperately need. People now consider sleep an obstacle. The phrase "I'll sleep when I'm dead" has become a motto for most workaholics and even social animals who want to make the most of their waking hours and then some. Why would they waste their time sleeping when they could just work for extra cash, spend time with friends, or catch up on their hobbies and interests because they don't get enough time for it during the day?

Depriving yourself of a good night's sleep on a regular basis depletes your energy levels in the long run. Whether it is staying out late with friends or scrolling through your social media all through the night, your body loses the ability to get a good night's sleep. Moreover, most of these activities leave your mind thinking and overthinking about your place in the universe and what you are doing with your life. Watching social media feeds of others going out and living life to the fullest or hearing from your friends how they are making the most out of their lives can leave you in a state of depression and anxiety.

IN THE PALE BLUE SCREENLIGHT

How often do you get ready to go to bed and turn your lights off only to reach for your cell phone and keep scrolling away with your head at an awkward angle. Don't worry, we have all been there. Though we can overlook the fact that you may be reading this page at night before heading off to sleep, why don't take in some useful information while you are here and perhaps you may just turn your phone off once you're done.

Our brain is much like any machine, and like any machine it runs the risk of being overtaxed if we continue using it all the time. The brain goes through several stages and processes while we sleep that are crucial to allow us to function fully during our waking hours. Nowadays, the smartphone has become an part of our lives so much that we cannot imagine life without it. It is also vital to have time away from that device so that our brain can get the rest that it deserves.

Several studies have found that overuse of smartphones can be hazardous to overall health, particularly before going to bed. The most critical reason is one you've likely heard of, and that is the blue light emitted by phone screens. This light in dark conditions is not only harmful to your eyes, but it also restricts the production of melatonin in your body. As we discussed in the previous chapter, melatonin is a hormone that regulates our sleep-wake cycle, or the circadian rhythm. It has been observed that our circadian rhythm is especially sensitive to blue light because of its short wavelength which can disrupt our sleep patterns drastically.

Of course, the blue light is just the physical manifestation of the problem. It is also what you see on the screen that keeps you up and alert, possibly even hyperalert as you see social media posts that you strongly agree or disagree with. Or even a comment thread that you simply must view all of to keep track of the argument, despite it having nothing to do with you. It could even be a strongly worded email from work that you received late at night that has unnerved you and you spend the whole night worrying over. This can leave you tense all the way until morning when you head out to work. Even if the content isn't too engrossing or engaging, your mind can wonder at the possibilities available to you, thanks to the internet. It could be late-night online shopping or playing random video games with total strangers from all around the world. In any case, your brain is all fired up and ready to pounce at the next screen swipe.

With all that physical and mental activity throughout the night, your mornings will see you more sluggish and tired, possibly uninterested in everything that is happening around you. Your eyes will be blinking constantly and you might even feel like your head is in a haze, which means that your alertness is severely diminished and not enough for you to exert all your energy for the day. Overtime, doing this can lead to a significant chronic sleep deficiency as well as an impression of you that is constantly tired and inefficient in the eyes of the people you interact with throughout the day. And who can blame them? The lack of concentration and interest can quickly become apparent in your work and tasks.

Staying up late also causes problems related to your physical health. Using a smartphone in the late hours while your body is looking for a chance to doze off can cause issues such as blurred vision, as well as fatigue and pain in the wrists, fingers, or neck (Kwon, Lee, et al., 2013). It also causes behavioral or mental problems such as interfering with education or work, reducing real-life social interactions, difficulties in maintaining relationships, and other maladaptive behavioral difficulties (Kuss & Griffiths, 2011).

Studies conducted with separate controlled groups, one which used smartphones regularly and one that did not, showed that people overusing their smartphones were more likely to experience anxiety and depression (Hwang, Yoo & Cho, 2012). As a result, technologically advanced societies are facing a serious public health problem in the form of poor sleep quality (Cheung & Wong, 2011), largely because of the use of the internet that is leading to insomnia and poor sleep quality, especially in adolescents (Lam, 2014). By the same token, another study suggests that depression and sleep-related problems were correlated with internet addiction in adolescents (Song et al, 2010).

Because our modern lives have become so dependent on the internet and smartphones, it is inconceivable that we will simply abandon our phones just like that before going to bed. Nevertheless, that is exactly what we have to do, though there are some tips as to how you can ease yourself into a phone-free sleep. As a rule, stop using any electronic devices at least 30 minutes before going to bed. This includes phones, tablets, computers, TVs, and even your smartwatches. This is a recommendation by the National Sleep Foundation, a non-profit involved in evidence-based and medically reviewed sleep research. Make it a habit every time you go to sleep to take a book with you to bed instead. Not only will you find yourself easing into a good sleep, but you will also feel more refreshed and energized the next day.

Of course, your phone will stay on while you sleep. So make sure that it is put on silent mode before you go to bed. Turn off Wi-Fi and data or simply turn on the "airplane mode" to ignore any kind of communication. All your phone should be able to alert you for is your morning wake-up alarm. If you don't do this, your phone can still receive alerts such as texts, social media updates, email alerts, game notifications, and so on that actually interrupt your deep sleep. You will constantly be triggered by your phone buzzing next to your pillow or on your nightstand and worse still, you may even be tempted to check what is happening. Before you know it, you are caught in it again, and such long-term disruptions to your sleep can reduce your total amount of REM sleep.

Should you need to take drastic measures, you may want to consider putting your phone in a different part of the room as far away from your bed as you can. Even better, consider putting your phone in a different room, whether it's the kitchen, the living room, the bathroom, even the basement if you have one. You can buy an alarm clock to ensure that you wake-up on time. Doing this will make it more unlikely that you will get up at odd hours of the night to check your phone, so your body is allowed to rest up for the next day. Most smartphones allow you to add a list of callers to be excluded from the vibrate mode. This way, you can rest assured that you won't miss an emergency call.

LET THERE BE DARK

One of the most important factors affecting our sleep is the overall lighting of the room where we sleep. Most people can intuitively sleep in the dark; however, there is a more complicated relationship between lighting and our sleep patterns. This relationship has also evolved a great deal since the invention of the electric light and its evolution from light bulbs, to fluorescent tubes, energy savers, and LED lights.

Although our biology dictates that our sleep patterns follow those of sunlight and darkness, we live in a time where light is surrounding us constantly. Gone are the days where people would sleep next to a campfire or under the stars after blowing out a lantern. Now, electric lighting is everywhere, from streetlights to billboards, from office lighting to electronic devices; the number of dark spaces is very limited wherever you go.

It has already been established that light plays a crucial role in regulating our circadian rhythm as well as the production of melatonin, both important factors to our state of alertness and state of rest. Our circadian rhythm is basically a 24-hour internal clock responsible for managing a wide range of internal processes within the body. Sleep is one of those processes and this rhythm is controlled by the circadian pacemaker, a small part of the brain.

This pacemaker is greatly influenced by exposure to light as soon as it enters the eye. From there, special cells on the retina sense it and carry it to the brain which interprets it as information about the time of day. The brain then sends signals throughout the body to operate under the conditions based on the time of day that the light has indicated. This is an appropriate response when we are exposed to only natural light, as our circadian rhythm is in sync with the sunrise and sunset to keep us awake during the day and asleep at night.

But what happens when our circadian pacemaker is overwhelmed by the constant sources of artificial lighting, especially at night? By receiving a steady stream of light exposure throughout the evening, our sleep cycle is affected so that we head for bed much later than we should. If we limit our exposure to artificial light in the nighttime, we go to bed earlier. The effects on our circadian rhythm vary as to the type of light and the amount of exposure as well as the time. Regardless of longer or shorter periods, any exposure to artificial light affects the circadian rhythm in the long term. It could be poorly timed exposure to artificial light or an excess amount of it, but your circadian rhythm is bound to be misaligned with the time of day and night.

Because of this, you will have little to no control over your sleep schedule which can lead to other health concerns. Aside from exhaustion and fatigue, you can also face irregular metabolism as well as weight gain, or worse still, an increased chance of cancer or cardiovascular problems. It also affects our mental health and mood as we have seen from the previous chapter, particularly in the regions with shorter days in winter and people facing Seasonal Affective Disorder (SAD).

Sleep can be affected by virtually all types of light but with varying impact. To measure in numbers, direct sunlight has up to 10,000 lux, which is far more intense than the brightest of office lighting that can reach only about 500 lux. Some artificial lighting has more illuminance and brightness depending on their utility, such as spotlights or floodlights, but it is an established fact that they also have a different wavelength when they are interpreted by the eye and the brain. For instance, many electronic devices such as smartphones, tablets, and laptops contain LED screens that emit a blue light. This blue light has a short wavelength and has a greater effect on melatonin and circadian rhythm. And as we saw above, extensive exposure to blue light in darker environments contributes greatly to sleep problems.

To elaborate further, exposure to light also affects melatonin which is naturally made in conjunction with light. The pineal gland in the brain begins melatonin production in response to darkness, but this is slowed down or halted whenever the light exposure is higher due to artificial lighting. Higher levels of melatonin facilitate sleep by increasing drowsiness as well as scheduling a proper sleep-wake cycle by normalizing the circadian rhythm. On average, we go through four to six sleep cycles of 70 to 120 minutes each. These cycles include both REM and non-REM sleep. But prolonged exposure to light can derail the transitions between our sleep cycles as we wake up repeatedly. This reduces our overall quality of sleep and length of restorative sleep stages.

People who frequently travel to international destinations also suffer from a misaligned circadian rhythm due to a disorder commonly known as jet lag. Normally, jet lag occurs after hopping five or more time zones because our body is still oriented to the city where we took off from. Imagine leaving a city in the day and spending hours upon hours in a plane only to land at a destination where the sun is still shining down at you. Such a condition can completely throw your circadian rhythm out of balance and you may face excessive daytime sleepiness, not getting the proper sleep because of the time of day, and so on. The only way to come out of the effects of jet lag is by acclimatizing to the new time zone which can take anywhere from several days to a couple of weeks.

A very common situation that causes circadian disorder is known as the shift work disorder. This is particularly for people working in occupations that have multiple shifts or even operate 24 hours a day. This includes hospitals, airports, call centers, law enforcement agencies, truck stops, hospitality centers such as hotels, and restaurant and diner chains. Most people may work evening or night shifts regularly or on a rotating schedule. It is estimated by the Bureau of Labor and Statistics that around 16% of American workers have late shifts such as evening or overnight. Aside from that, most high-achieving professionals such as business owners and executives are known to work long hours, possibly sleeping in the office itself and may even have employees staying late to work on critical and time-sensitive projects.

Because of working in the later hours, shift workers have to sleep during the daytime which affects their circadian rhythm a great deal. Furthermore, this creates an environment where a person is exposed to light at times when the body realizes that it should be dark, and such a disruption in circadian rhythm ultimately leads to shift work disorder which can cause a lack of sufficient sleep or excessive sleepiness, altered moods, lack of focus at work, and even workplace accidents or embarrassments.

Ideally, sleep should be an activity that is done at night. When you close your eyes, your mind begins to go into a shut-down mode and that allows it to rest up and be energized for the next day. Pitch-black darkness is a very conducive environment for the best kind of sleep as it minimizes potential disruptions to sleep or any other distractions. Keeping a light on while sleeping, such as a night light, can interfere with your sleep cycles and create a fragmented sleeping experience. According to research, our eyelids are not enough to block out all forms of light, and even the tiniest bit of indoor light can find its way through our eyelids, ending up disrupting our circadian rhythm.

Aside from that, having a light source such as a night light, reading lamp, or a smartphone with blue light can cause other health concerns such as straining the eyes, irregular metabolism leading to weight gain, and even the risk of cancer. Ambient light during sleep even at low levels can strain our eyes resulting in soreness, tiredness, and general discomfort, not to mention difficulty in focusing. As for metabolism, our circadian rhythm can be so misaligned by any lights on during sleep that there is a greater risk of weight gain. A study shows that women who slept with a light or TV on could experience weight gain of up to ten pounds or more despite having sufficient control over their exercise and diet habits. And what is even worse is that, in some cases, this weight gain could occur without any disruption to sleep.

There is speculation that people with homes containing high levels of artificial night lighting have created an environment that could increase the risk of breast and prostate cancers according to one observational study. Nevertheless, further studies are required to completely confirm such a relation.

It would help a great deal if you set up your bedroom in such a way that you get the best sleep. How can you do that? Make it as dark as possible. Start off with blackout curtains that effectively block out external light which will create a darker environment. This is especially helpful if you live in apartment blocks that have lighting all around from billboards and street lights. Aside from that, using a small, low-powered night lamp instead of your room's main lights before going to sleep creates a calm and serene atmosphere for you to transition into sleep and darkness. Low lighting coupled with warm color temperature can work wonders with relaxation and may help you fall asleep.

Also, it cannot be stressed enough how important it is to minimize the presence of technology and devices in your room, especially those that have an LED screen and are connected to the internet. It would help if you keep them out of the room completely so that you aren't tempted to get out of bed to check any notifications you feel you are missing out on. Most smartphones now come with built-in night filters that alter the piercing blue light into a warmer, yellowish tint. This helps to reduce the stress on your eyes, though it still doesn't mean your mind isn't giving its full attention to the contents of your screen.

In some cases, having some kind of light on while sleeping is actually a necessity. Fear of the dark can affect anyone, no matter how old they are. Having some kind of light during sleep may provide them with some comfort. Nevertheless, it is recommended to keep night lights at the lowest settings or have night lights with a sleep timer that turn off after a certain time, by which you will have hopefully fallen asleep. Of course, it goes without saying that fear of the dark could reach serious extremes, in which case it is best to consult with a mental health professional.

A common reason to wake up at night is to visit the bathroom, which could be made difficult for children, older adults, and people with eyesight disorders such as night blindness. Having motion-sensor lights in hallways or corridors leading to the bathroom can help, or have a low-intensity light in the bathroom that turns on automatically whenever it detects motion. If you are married or live with a partner who has different preferences when it comes to the night light, their habits may actually prevent you from going to sleep in the dark. It could be because they watch TV or read with a night lamp. If this is the case, try to have a conversation with them about how distracting it is for you. On the other hand, you could wear a close-fitting eye mask that can completely black out any light.

UNDERSTAND YOUR CIRCADIAN RHYTHM

We have already gone into detail about how your circadian rhythm regulates and manages all the daily functions that your body performs based on a specific and choreographed routine. This routine is based on physical and chemical changes in your body in sync with the pattern of day and night. The circadian rhythm is hardwired genetically to influence your energy levels, alertness, and hunger, which helps you to feel your best when you follow a natural rhythm. Every person has their own unique and specific preferences or chronotypes that determine their particular alignment with the pattern of the sun.

For instance, your chronotype could be an "early bird" if you are more active in the morning and daytime, and conversely it could be a "night owl" if your schedule is attuned to the evening and night. This chronotype is determined based on certain factors such as core body temperature, melatonin levels, cortisol levels, and growth hormone. For early birds, your core body temperature drops by the time you reach your scheduled bedtime and rises again before the morning. Along with this, your melatonin levels will increase before your bedtime at night and cortisol rushes through your body to wake you up completely energized in the morning. Also, a large dose of growth hormone is released when you go to sleep so that it can carry out nighttime maintenance within your body. This happens when your circadian rhythm is properly aligned.

On the other hand, night owls see a drop in core body temperature roughly two or three hours after that of early birds and the same goes for the increase in melatonin levels. This pushes back their average sleep time and makes them feel restless even when it is well past their bedtime. Due to this, they may not get the rush of cortisol they need to jump start their day, and the function of the growth hormone may be impaired. According to research by chronobiologists, 40% of the population are early birds while 30% are night owls, with the remaining standing somewhere in between.

There are obvious health consequences to a misalignment in your circadian rhythm. Aside from hunger, tiredness, lack of concentration or focus, and constantly drifting off to sleep, a chronically misaligned circadian rhythm can have severe negative impacts on your critical internal processes, such as your immune system, gastrointestinal system, reproductive system, endocrine or hormone system, and cardiovascular system. Trying to get a full night's sleep may not be enough if you aren't going to bed at the optimal time based on your chronotype. It could affect the distribution of your sleep stages and affect deep and REM sleep.

Your circadian alignment also depends largely on the majority of society and their habits which make them early birds rather than night owls. Most businesses, services, and educational institutions see a vast majority of activity in the daytime starting bright and early in the morning. This makes it more favorably looked upon to be an early bird. This does put night owls at a disadvantage as their natural wake cycle does not align with the rest of their surroundings. Not to mention that night owls accrue a lot of missed hours of sleep that they cannot make up for. Even sleeping longer on weekends does not help and it shows in their overall performance.

Based on this, your ideal bedtime should be set to as early as possible to coincide with the sunset, and this way your body's circadian rhythm can be played out regardless of whether you want to sleep or not. Some of the positive signs of a healthy and aligned circadian rhythm are having a full seven to nine hours of sleep and being able to fall asleep in a short period of time; this can be anywhere from five to twenty minutes. A regular sleep schedule will prevent you from being restless through the night and reduce tossing and turning. You should also be getting 20% to 25% of REM sleep and 15% to 20% of deep sleep. And of course, you should be waking up completely well-rested, invigorated, and energized.

5

THE POWER OF MINDFULNESS PRACTICES

"Whatever the present moment contains, accept it as if you had chosen it. Always work with it, not against it."

— ECKHART TOLLE

D epression continues to be a major health concern for older adults, making them more socially isolated and unable to retain their cognitive function. Several treatments have been tried and tested to alleviate its symptoms. From psychotherapy to antidepressants, most medical front-line treatments are taken in reaction to a depressive episode. However, there is reason to believe that it can be proactively reduced in the long-term by engaging in regular meditation. The goal of such meditation is to alter the way your brain reacts to stress and anxiety, which can help you overcome depression more effectively.

In order for this to work, you will have to use your mind and willpower as your primary weapons against depression. To do so, you will have to train, or rather trick, your mind to be able to not respond negatively to any circumstances that may trigger depression. This can be achieved by mindfulness practices such as guided breathing to realign your body with your mind and brighten your mood.

Let's start with how your brain reacts to depression, particularly with its major triggers like experiences of stress and self-doubt. Scientists believe that people dealing with depression have a hyperactive medial prefrontal cortex (mPFC), a region of the brain that is largely known as the "me center." This is because the mPFC is where your mind processes the information about yourself, your goals, your dreams, and your concerns about past events and what to expect in the future. As most depression comes from situations where you question your earlier decisions or decisions regarding your future, your mPFC goes into overdrive, which we normally consider to be overthinking.

Aside from the mPFC, the amygdala is also a region of the brain linked to depression. Known as the "fear center," the amygdala is responsible for the fight-or-flight response and it triggers the release of cortisol from the adrenal glands in order to respond to any threats. Both the mPFC and the amygdala work off each other to trigger depression, as the former instantly reacts to stress and anxiety while the latter responds to any dangers that you may be foreseeing.

What meditation does is train the brain for sustained focus, and uses that focus to fight off any kind of negative thoughts, emotions, or physical sensations. It allows you to act with clarity upon perceiving any of the triggers of depression, and also helps to break the connection between the me center and the fear center. With sustained practice of meditation, you will be in a better position to ignore any negativity brought about by stress and anxiety, and will notice a drop in your stress levels immediately.

Meditation also helps to protect the hippocampus, an area of the brain that is involved in memory. A study has shown that people suffering from chronic depression tend to have a smaller hippocampus region which creates problems such as loss of the ability to create new memories. Moreover, a damaged or shrinking hippocampus can even lead to Alzheimer's disease. On the other hand, the study observed an increase in the volume of gray matter in the hippocampus among people who meditate for 30 minutes a day regularly, thus improving their memory retention.

WHAT MEDITATION ACTUALLY DOES

Many may think that meditation pushes stress aside and blocks out negativity. In truth, meditation actually helps you to notice these negative thoughts and makes sure that you understand that you do not have to act upon them. It helps you to exert your own control over the negativity that is aiming to trigger depression. It can be easily accomplished by simple mindfulness practices. This could include closing your eyes and repeating a word or phrase that you find reassuring and calming, inhaling, exhaling, and counting your breaths, or counting to a number allowing your heart rate to gradually slow down. Performing breathing exercises and mindfulness practices helps you to stay a reasonable distance away from the negativity. This provides you with enough time to understand your negative thoughts or emotions and consider a more appropriate course of action to address them.

Meditation and breathing exercises can also help you deal with anxiety. For instance, you could be stressed about going to a doctor's appointment or on a first date. This is where you will find yourself with a fast heart rate, cold and clammy hands, and a sweaty forehead. But meditating for a few moments before such an engagement can help your brain and body to properly deal with the stress response and remain calm.

Because of the complex nature of depression, you can be led towards dark thoughts while in a depressive state. By constantly and regularly practicing meditation, not only will you truly feel those negative emotions, but you will also reach a point where you will accept your depression for what it is.

More often than not, the thought of meditation to combat something like depression may be met with skepticism. It may sound as if someone is telling you to smile more or think positively whenever you feel down. Now, that doesn't mean that meditation will completely erase all the symptoms of depression, but it can make you more adept at managing them. For one thing, it will change your response to all the negative thoughts of being hopeless, worthless, or angry at yourself or the way things are going for you.

At the onset, meditation can actually increase your awareness of such thoughts and experiences, which may make it sound like a counterproductive practice. However, meditation actually helps you to be attentive to those thoughts and feelings without becoming too harsh or critical of yourself. It teaches you the truth: Things will not always go your way and the way you respond to them will either make or break you. You will learn not to ignore or push away these thoughts and feelings. Only by accepting them can we let them go and move on. This practice of acceptance helps to disrupt the hold negativity has over us without being too judgmental of ourselves.

For instance, think about your position in life as it is and look for the moments that make your life worth living. You feel the happiness and love from your friends and loved ones and are more accepting of your life. That is, until you entertain the notion that maybe you don't deserve to have such a good life. Instead of letting that thought overwhelm you with sadness, you can start meditating. Then you will be able to acknowledge that it is just one possibility out of many. There are more possibilities that are actually in your favor. Instead of perceiving yourself as undeserving or worthless, you can let this thought pass through your awareness by meditating and letting it float by like a leaf floating down the river. The more you poke and prod at the leaf with a stick, the likelier it is to sink.

Using this method, you will learn to stay present in the moment. This will help you notice the warning signs of a possible depressive episode before it arrives. This way, you can learn how to effectively manage your depression and how to easily pay attention to your emotions. The next time you find yourself experiencing increased irritability and unease because of a shift in thought patterns, you could simply focus on meditation and self-care in order to keep things on a positive note. A depressive episode may manifest itself in ways such as loss of interest in your favorite activities, loss of focus, loss of appetite, or other tell-tale signs of depression we have reviewed previously.

Furthermore, recent research has shown that mindfulness-based cognitive therapy can help with lowering the chances of going into depression, particularly if it is a chronic depression. This therapy is a variation of psychotherapy that includes mindfulness meditation practices that can help to reduce the effects and symptoms of depression once you incorporate them into your regular life. Much like long-term medication, meditative practices need to be continued on a daily basis to provide the best results for your mental health. Think of it as exercise for your mind that fights off the depressive tendencies and thoughts.

HOW TO MEDITATE MINDFULLY

Incorporating meditative practices into your daily routine is not that difficult, despite it appearing to be a bit odd in the beginning. Thinking of meditation may bring images of deeply meditating monks; however, meditation is actually not that complicated. In most cases, learning proper meditation starts off with sitting down and getting comfortable. Then again, meditation can also be performed while standing up or lying down. As long as you find the position comfortable and unburdening. Keeping your eyes closed is also helpful as it keeps external distractions at bay.

Next, take deep, slow breaths through your nose. As you do, pay close attention to your breathing, including how it feels to inhale and exhale, as well as the sound of your breaths. It is completely normal for your thoughts to wander away from your breath; however, you must catch yourself and bring your focus right back to your breathing. Paying attention to how your breaths feel and sound helps us to remember exactly what we are focusing on.

From your breaths, start to shift your attention to the other parts of your body. Think of this as a body scan where you focus on different parts of the body and shift your attention all over to find out if there is any stress or pressure on them. Most people like to begin with their feet and move up, while others start with their hands or head and move towards the rest of the body in sequence. The goal here is to focus your awareness on your body as you move from one part to the next while continuing to breathe in and out. With each of your deep breaths, you can note how each part of your body feels simply by thinking about it. For instance, if you start with your feet, focus on if there is any pain or tension in your toes, heels, soles, or ankles.

Assuming that you do notice something problematic such as an ache or tension, you can start a visualization exercise to help curb this sensation. This works by imagining your breaths being directed to the part of the body that is in pain. These breaths will have a relaxing and soothing effect on that body part as you picture those tight muscles loosening. You can imagine in your mind's eye how that pain is gradually decreasing with each of your breaths focusing on that body part or parts. You will begin to feel comfortable with your bodily sensations. This will help you become attuned to the changes as they come up. Once you complete your body scan from head to toe, you can bring your focus back solely to your breathing. Take as much time as you need to become comfortable and relaxed. The body scan will help you identify the areas of tension. Master this, and you will be able to relieve them.

The next stage involves dealing with any unwanted or unpleasant thoughts and emotions that may arise as you continue to breathe. It is time to acknowledge their existence, albeit briefly, and then turn your attention back to your breathing. Remember that your attention will wander from your breathing, no matter if you are a newbie at meditation or have been practicing for many years. Nevertheless, as long as you can bring your focus back to your breathing and meditation, you will be able to create a better awareness and more compassion for yourself.

The body scan described above is one of many ways with which you can meditate. There are no right or wrong methods. You may find certain methods to be effective for you but they may not be as effective for someone else. The results can be mixed, and therefore it never hurts to seek out help by taking a class or having a meditation coach. There are many guided meditations available online that are both free and paid; you can also add your own creative spin to meditation so long as it keeps you internally satisfied.

There are some habits that you can incorporate to make you better at your meditation techniques. For instance, practice at the same time regularly and start small before gradually increasing. No amount of time is too small, even five minutes a day at a suitable time can work wonders. Then, as you find yourself becoming more focused, increase your time to ten minutes and then fifteen minutes and so on. And there is no limit to where you can do it, so long as you are in a comfortable position. It could be in the shower where you perform a body scan every morning, sitting down at your workstation before you start and get attuned to your surroundings, or even before going to bed each night. The key here is to try out various scenarios before you find your sweet spot for meditation, and this way you are likely to stick to it.

Another crucial element to meditation is developing and using your own mantra. You may think this sounds corny, but it is actually a very effective tool to keep your thoughts from straying away into unwanted and unpleasant territory. And let's not forget that your thoughts will wander no matter how hard you try, but with a mantra you can refocus your thoughts. The mantra could be a simple word or a phrase that you can repeat during your meditative exercise, and it is something you are both comfortable with and confident about. It could be a humming sound to help you breathe more clearly, or a phrase that helps you feel calm. It could be something that you remember affectionately or has a deeper meaning for you.

Examples of these could be "I am calm," "I am free," "It's all good," "All will be well," and so on.

You also don't have to be boxed within four walls to effectively meditate. Though the goal is to minimize outside influence, going out for a walk in the park or sitting outside on a bench can actually provide much-needed stimulation for your meditation, not to mention a fresh supply of oxygen for you to breathe in. This might be the case if you do not feel like being cooped up inside and would rather be outdoors among nature. This is actually because nature can provide a completely serene environment such as fresh air and soothing sounds that can help you calm our mind, and also help your overall health. You could also add some intense activity such as running or exercising, particularly if you are an active person. Doing some interval training or jumping jacks will allow you to keep your arms, legs, and other active body parts in a repetetive motion.

Don't forget that meditation requires a lot of practice, effort, and time. If you go into this believing that you need to feel a huge difference instantly, then you may need to reconsider the whole idea behind meditation. Alternatively, you should start by noticing small and gradual improvements over time as you focus on meditation, taking things one at a time. A lot of research monitors the impact of meditation over many weeks, or even months, as it is a regular practice that needs to be continued on a daily basis. This is important if you wish to see a gradual and significant reduction in your levels of depression. That doesn't mean that you won't feel any improvements after first starting this practice. Focus on the positive changes that become apparent such as an improvement in your overall mood or your focus at work and on other tasks.

Also keep in mind that meditation is only one of many approaches to help reduce depression, but nothing can truly cure you of depression. Most therapists will recommend meditation as part of a larger treatment, depending on the intensity and frequency of your depressive episodes. Keep in mind that it has its limits. This is especially true when dealing with a major depressive episode. A nervous breakdown may indicate underlying depression or anxiety. As was mentioned earlier, meditation often brings you face-to-face with your negative thoughts, but these could also be too overwhelming for meditation alone to handle.

Under those circumstances, it is recommended to seek immediate counseling from a mental health professional, especially if you notice a significant decrease in your quality of life as well as a struggle to manage your daily responsibilities. Furthermore, you may experience pain, fatigue, loss of appetite, and worse still, you may be lashing out at others and contemplating self-harm or even suicide. And though meditation may help you try to escape those thoughts, you should not rely wholly on it, especially if these thoughts become chronic.

SELF-LOVE AND ATTENTION

One of the things meditation helps us focus on is being more appreciative of who we are as a person and also to show some love, care, and affection to ourselves. By providing this much attention to our very beings, we focus on the most important relationship in our lives, and that is with ourselves. We may show love to ourselves by rewarding our sense of achievement or general good mood by treating ourselves to a nice dinner or a present such as clothes or a trip to a day spa. In other cases, we react too harshly, judgmentally, or are overly critical when we fall short of our expectations or fail in achieving our goals. At this stage, we begin to punish ourselves by berating ourselves or taking the blame for all of our perceived shortcomings.

It is important to realize that we also need to show ourselves some love and care at the times we need it the most, particularly when we fall short of our goals. By assuring ourselves that we are not disappointed with our own efforts and can strive to try harder the next time, we feel a sense of personal growth, stronger motivation, and a higher level of satisfaction that leads towards building a healthier mindset. It isn't an easy undertaking; practicing self-love requires a great deal of deprogramming from our earlier state of self-deprecation, and this requires a great deal of patience, practice, and belief in ourselves.

You can actually practice self-love immediately by creating a routine around yourself to focus on your goals and achievements. For starters, you can create a vision board that is a physical manifestation to visualize your goals. You can do this by gathering small items and placing them on a board that you can see every day. These items could be anything such as quotations, verses, photographs, artwork, totems or icons, magazine clippings, and so on. All of these things can trigger motivation as well as a positive mindset in order for you to focus on achieving your goals. Seeing these items over and over again on a daily basis helps you to not just identify your end goals, but also to work out the methods by which you can achieve them. If an item on your vision board represents a promotion, then you have to visualize in your mind the steps needed to achieve that goal. The vision board helps you to get in the right frame of mind as well as identify the path to take, and it provides much-needed clarity to the process.

You can also learn more about personality types to get an idea about how to become more compassionate towards yourself. Learning more and more details about the kind of person you are and what you are capable of helps you to appreciate your uniqueness and tap into your abilities, skills, and personal qualities that will help you to get ahead. For example, if you have an introverted nature then you might be pushing down your introvert tendencies just to fit into an environment where extroverts thrive. However, you need to embrace your introverted nature and recognize what makes you unique in this world. There are things that only you are capable of and that sets you apart from the rest.

It isn't just enough that you love your inner self. You must learn to love your outer self as well. The more you care about your body and appreciate how you look, the better you will feel about yourself from within. Radiating an image of confidence and positivity can also be manifested physically by exercising and letting your body become fit and strong. Simple exercises such as yoga or interval training outdoors can help you build a strong foundation to build your personality both inside and out. Working out can be more effective if you do it outdoors in nature. It helps you to quickly navigate away from negative energy and feel much better about yourself as you do it. Green spaces are highly conducive and invigorating as they let you free yourself from your existing burdens, not to mention the fresh air and sunlight do wonders for your body.

And if you really want to show yourself some love, why not say it with a heartfelt message? It could be in the form of a letter, an email, or a text. Write about a positive quality you admire in yourself, or an achievement that you are proud of. More often than not, we write all sorts of praise for people we love and admire, such as our friends, family, and peers. The same amount of admiration needs to be shown for yourself, if not more. It will also help you reflect on all the aspects that you have thought of and become more motivated with what you have set out to accomplish in the future.

You should also check in with your inner self more often and find the voice that you hear every day. Your inner voice tells you many things that you may need to get through the day. A great deal of this could be positive reinforcement and affirmations. So you have to check your tone with how you respond to yourself, particularly to be more positive, encouraging, forgiving, empowering, and above all else, kind. Such inner dialogue is crucial for you to support your journey towards self-love. It will also help to switch to something more positive if you feel that negative thoughts are gaining the upper hand. For example, if you make an error or mistake, instead of regretting it and blaming yourself for your inefficiencies, focus on how you can learn from this mistake and talk to yourself about what you would do differently next time to achieve more positive results.

6

GIVE MORE TIME TO YOURSELF

"When you say 'yes' to others, make sure you are not saying 'no' to yourself."

— PAULO COELHO

Think back to before COVID-19 became a full-blown pandemic and remember how life was at that point. We were constantly moving, never staying in the same place, never having time for ourselves or the people we cared about. We were spreading ourselves thin; being everything to everyone and in that we forgot about ourselves as people and individuals. Then the pandemic hit, and with it came lockdowns and self-isolating practices that put everyone at home. This led to a grave effect on everyone's mental health as people began to worry about everything they possibly could. Whether it was the fear of the virus itself or the restrictions in place that kept them indoors, not being able to go back to school as usual, or being worried about where the next paycheck was going to come from. The pandemic has taken its toll.

However, this sort of vacation from the world has made people look inward at themselves and discover all the things about themselves that they have either willfully ignored or haven't been able to pay attention to in their busy schedules. And, if for nothing else than to have something to do, everyone has started to look for ways to be more productive or creative. Many are searching for how they can achieve self-improvement. Establishing a routine can help people feel a sense of structure in their lives. The World Health Organization (WHO) has recommended having a regular pattern of eating, sleeping, hygiene, and exercise in order to look after your mental health. And as we are talking about routines, hobbies are something that can be done on a regular basis that not only provide comfort in these trying times, but can also be fun to do.

Engaging in hobbies helps people ease feelings of depression as these activities are nourishing to the heart and soul. Using your skills or learning a new one can feel both rewarding and delightful. You might be interested in improving your art skills, learning to knit, to cook, or how to play a musical instrument. There are plenty of do-it-yourself (DIY) kits and guides that will keep you engaged and feeling productive. The satisfaction one gets from creating something out of nothing or letting their imagination run wild is a powerful deterrent to depressive and negative thoughts.

It may make you wonder just why you never took up a hobby in the first place, or why you didn't continue one as you grew older. Most people have at one point or another had a hobby they loved to do, particularly in their childhood or adolescent years. Then, the burdens of education and work turned into the singular driving force in their lives. Because of the strain of academic and professional pursuits, people stop taking time out for themselves and no longer enrich their souls using their creativity. Ask anyone if they like reading books, and the answer you are likely to get is that they don't get enough time to read. This is actually a symptom of depression known as anhedonia, which is losing interest and joy in the things that you actually enjoyed doing for yourself. Imagine being so depressed that you stop doing something you're truly passionate about.

This could be anything from reading colorful comic books to creating vibrant oil paintings.

Unfortunately, there is no medication that can alleviate the symptom of anhedonia; it is one that the majority of patients with depression would most like to be free of. The only logical solution to this is to make the time for your interests and pleasures. The lockdown has provided ample opportunity for people to do so, and even doctors have been known to ask patients with mild to moderate depression to take up a hobby in lieu of antidepressants.

HOW HOBBIES HELP

There is virtually no limit to the kind of hobbies you can take up from the comfort of your own home and with limited supplies. With the wave of eco-friendly and green living on the rise, many people have taken to gardening using small clay pots or even by reusing old plastic bottles. That combines the joy of both gardening and creating a DIY solution, plus it also reduces the amount of plastic waste being discarded irresponsibly. Taking it a step further, water from air conditioning exhaust can be used to water the plants, and it is actually better for plants because it is chlorine-free. And with an activity like gardening, it is actually rewarding as you invest yourself in an actual living being's growth. Watching a plant grow and blossom over time brings its own sense of joy and accomplishment.

The above highlights how putting in such efforts and getting a result triggers the reward system in our brains. We feel pleasure in achieving something such as taking care of a plant because chemical neurotransmitters such as dopamine are released. These are basically feel-good chemicals; they help us feel pleasure at achieving something which helps to reduce the symptoms of depression. The same goes for other hobbies as well, such as improving our physical health through exercising or changing to a new diet, creating an amazing painting or handicraft, or being entranced by playing a musical instrument. It also follows a form of psychological treatment called behavioral action which helps people to overcome their depression by scheduling in time for their hobbies.

The feeling of pleasure and achievement isn't the only reason to take up regular hobbies. There are benefits to overall health as well. For instance, reading both fiction and non-fiction can help you improve your knowledge, vocabulary, and perhaps even prompt you to have a crack at writing yourself. Regular exercise can help you improve your physical fitness and improve your mental health. Some research has shown that playing board games, doing puzzles, reading books, and playing musical instruments help you to improve your memory and attention to detail. This can actually reduce the possibility of dementia as you grow older.

Some occupations such as essential services require people to continue to venture out into the world, even in a pandemic landscape. But those who are working should also spend time on their hobbies in order to unwind from their daily routines. Hobbies can help to reduce stress and anxiety, and are genuine mood-lifters whether it is doing something outdoors or indoors. Doing something creative like art or music keeps your mind stimulated as you seek to improve after each and every milestone. Beyond the pandemic, if you are into group activities such as sports and games, this is a great opportunity for you to socialize and improve your communication skills with your friends and peers, not to mention have a great deal of fun.

Ideally, our interests vary from academic, educational, creative, physical, athletic, health-related, or even something unique to you. These could be done either individually or in a group. Social media has made it far easier to connect with other like-minded hobbyists. Groups on social media help people to showcase their talents by sharing their artwork, music, writings, and so on. They are also great places to get suggestions and feedback about your work, as well as find inspiration and learn something new.

Some hobbyists are actually anxious and skeptical about sharing their own creations with others. They fear they may be judged for being too amateurish or not as good as most of the others in the group. But what they don't realize is that everyone has had a journey towards reaching their skill levels. If you have the confidence to share your work, it will only help you grow. If nothing else, you can get pointers and encouragement from everyone to work on your talents. Even just watching what others are doing can help your confidence grow enough that you can create something on your own. And sooner or later, you will be sharing your creativity with the world!

Find a hobby that resonates with you or makes you feel good. If you are starting something for the first time, start with something you feel you can easily learn. Focus on the basics. Most hobbies, such as music, offer beginner exercises that are easy to understand and pick up. Music provides several health benefits for your mental health as it helps you manage your emotions and stress. It also provides an outlet to express your feelings in the genre of your choice, whether it is something upbeat such as jazz or sad such as the blues. Furthermore, it can be a great way to connect with a large group, as most people find music touching for the soul. That is a kind of connection that will enrich you spiritually as well.

BENEFITS OF PHYSICAL ACTIVITIES

Playing sports is another great way to ward off depressive thoughts and negativity. These help you to keep yourself physically active and increase blood flow. You'll feel more relaxed afterwards. Staying active also enhances the flow of hormones that help you feel happy about yourself and your well-being. You will have noticed that athletes are some of the happiest people out there and that is because of how well they feel after they perform. Furthermore, any time they are sidelined or not able to perform due to injury is when they feel at their lowest, because they do not get to enjoy the thrill of the sport.

This is because regular physical activity raises your level of endorphins and serotonin, which greatly benefits your self-esteem. These endorphins trigger a positive and pleasant feeling in the body that acts similar to morphine. They interact with the receptors in your brain by acting as analgesics and sedatives. These are released as a response to neurotransmitters in your brain. Endorphins are produced in your brain, spinal cord, and other parts of your body, and they bind with neuron receptors that also bind with some pain reducers such as morphine. The best part about endorphins is that they do not lead to any addiction or dependence as morphine does to some people.

Sports and physical activity help people find a sense of bliss or joy. The term "runner's high" or "jogger's high" represents just that: A feeling of euphoria while running or jogging that helps you get a satisfying feeling as well as a sense of re-energizing and positivity. Exercising, intense workouts, and practicing sports regularly has been proven to stave off the symptoms of depression and anxiety. It also improves physical fitness which also couples with an invigorated self-esteem, and improves your sleep. The endorphins responsible for giving you a "feel-good" rush also improve your concentration and sharpen you mentally for any tasks you may have. They also stimulate the growth of new brain cells which are key to preventing age-related memory decline.

By maintaining a habit of exercising, you are investing in your mind, body, and soul. This will result in an improved sense of self-worth. You will feel strong and powerful, and see that you are physically manifesting those traits. Scheduled exercises in the morning or afternoon, even in short bursts, can help to regulate your sleep patterns. Meditation and other relaxing exercises such as yoga or stretching before you go to bed can help you get better sleep at night. Furthermore, all exercise promotes better blood flow and it leads to greater cardiovascular health. Your heart rate will increase when you exercise, and you will improve your endurance and feel relaxed once you stop, leaving you more energized.

Exercise also helps to build resilience against the mental or emotional challenges that life throws at you as you work on yourself rather than drown out your sorrows in negative behaviors such as social withdrawal or substance abuse. Therefore, regular physical activity impacts your overall health by strengthening your heart, boosting your energy levels, managing your blood pressure, improving your muscle tone and strength, reducing body fat, making bones stronger, and so on. And let's not forget that exercising outdoors with appropriate sun protection helps us stock up on our vitamin D levels!

The best part is that any kind of physical exercise is good for managing depression. Even moderate exercise such as biking, jogging, low-impact aerobics, tennis, swimming, gardening or yard work, yoga, and dancing can help us feel more relaxed and energized once we are done. Doing it with a partner, spouse, friends, and even your own children can prove to be beneficial as it becomes a group activity that will not only benefit your physical health, it will also provide you with emotional comfort and support from those around you.

The thrill of physical activity causes an instant blood rush that positively affects your brain function, particularly to help with mental illnesses. It can be used both as a standalone or combined treatment with medication and therapy. It does not have the same stigma attached to it as being on antidepressants or seeing a therapist or counselor. But do keep in mind that every person has their own path to recovery and a healthy balance between physical exercise and talking about your feelings with a professional can go a long way towards managing depression. Plus it also reduces the risk of cognitive decline in adults and the elderly. Studies have shown a risk reduction of 20% to 30% for developing dementia in adults who took up exercise and other physical activities.

It has also been observed that physical exercise is capable of reducing depression and anxiety in children, adolescents, and teens. Schools that have regular physical education classes and other sports opportunities in outdoor or open spaces can help to improve cognitive performance and reduce the symptoms related to anxiety and attention deficit disorder. A study published in the Journal of

Adolescent Health observed that students in grades 8 to 12 have less stress and better mental health when they play team sports such as basketball, soccer, track and field, wrestling, and gymnastics. Such students also showed better scores on post-graduation mental health assessments three years after graduating, as opposed to those students who did not engage in any team sports.

The study concluded that playing sports during adolescence is linked to reduced depression symptoms and perceived stress, and better mental health overall. This goes to show that physical activities from the ages of 12 to 17 provided several benefits such as more confidence, sharper focus and alertness, reduced levels of stress and tension, improved cognitive function, better ability to cope with stress, enhanced critical thinking and judgment skills, and better quality of life.

Depression can also be linked to Post Traumatic Stress Disorder (PTSD) and trauma which is characterized by an immobilization stress response to a traumatic event. A traumatic event could be witnessing a car crash, a violent attack, or the death of a loved one. A person could experience long-term trauma during childhood or while in an abusive relationship. This, as well as isolated incidents, can lead to the development of PTSD. With physical activities such as exercise, you can do cross-lateral movements that engage both arms and legs. By being regularly active, you are able to focus on your body moving and becoming unstuck from the sense of trauma that you may be experiencing. Other activities such as rock climbing, hiking, sailing, whitewater rafting, skiing, skydiving, sailing, and so on, have a significant impact on reducing the symptoms of PTSD.

QUALITY TIME WITH FRIENDS

You will have realized by this point that doing activities to enrich yourself and give you a sense of euphoria and accomplishment is amplified even more when it can be shared with friends. The chances of having good and stable mental health are increased when you are among others who you love spending time with and you can share happiness, laughter, and joy with them. People with positive energy tend to transmit it to others, and therefore you have a unique opportunity to bond and vibe at the same frequency with others. This greatly helps you to have a more positive experience and outlook on life.

Moreover, as humans are social creatures, we don't do well when we are totally by ourselves and have no one in our orbit. It's important to have friends that we can share a joke with, have a nice chat over dinner or drinks, or just hang out and play video games with.

Spending quality time with our friends can greatly help us to develop trust and confidence in others which contributes significantly to our mental health.

Of course, this is further complicated when we are caught up in our busy schedules or stuck at home due to the lockdown restrictions. Finding time to do things with our friends is often put on the backburner as we prioritize other commitments such as work, education, and even romantic relationships. Even social media, the modern marvel that endeavored to bring friends together, has actually pushed them apart. Why go through all the trouble of dressing up and going out to meet friends when you can simply have a video call or chat with them on instant messaging instead?

Spending actual face-to-face time with friends is vital for one's mental well-being. By doing so, we are able to talk about our feelings and build trust. Staying in touch allows us to bond with those who we feel a kinship for. It offers opportunities to care and support others if they are going through a difficult time or are experiencing mental health issues. Helping someone to combat their own stress and anxiety by being there and listening to them will help them feel better about themselves. In this way, you can find some comfort and self-worth within yourself.

You may have noticed that you grow detached when you are under a cloud of depression or mental illness. Such feelings can make you unsure of taking part in social events, as you believe you will not be able to immerse yourself in the experience. You may find yourself feeling out of place or be intimidated by the presence of everyone having a good time, and it will actually become apparent to the others. Oftentimes, friends feel that your mental health problems may be keeping you isolated and withdrawn, in which case they are not completely able to understand what you may be going through. Worse still, they may not be able to say the right things or respond in the manner that will help you reduce your anxiety.

Because of this, you may feel that you are losing friends while you are struggling with your mental health problems. This can make you feel lonely, isolated, and hopeless. Now, reverse the roles where someone you know may also be suffering from a mental illness and you may be struggling to help them, not even knowing where to start. That can also be a daunting proposition. Regardless of who is facing the illness, it is important to stay in touch and maintain those friendships, as well as having a sense of what they might be going through. Talking to them, trying to understand what they feel, suggesting solutions such as therapy and exercise, and above all else, being there for them can go a long way to bring them out of their shell and back into the world ready to face their challenges.

Now, revert the roles back to you, and tell your friends what you feel, how you would like to feel, and what they can do to help you.

Spending time with friends is not only important for your mental health, but it also applies to other aspects of your life. Their presence can also help you to avoid negative behaviors like smoking or drug and alcohol abuse. They can also help you make positive lifestyle choices not just limited to food and exercise. You can approach friends for suggestions for anything, whether it is a recommendation for a restaurant or a new smartphone, or advice on which investment opportunities to go for. Research shows that friends who spend quality time together can influence each other's lifestyle behaviors. Good friends can help you make positive choices, especially when you aren't sure what to do and need advice.

Friendships also become instrumental when you are facing insecurities or doubts. It is then that their counsel can help you examine your options from a different point of view. It's always a good idea to get a second opinion over any major decisions that you may be facing. Counting on your friends when you feel uncertain means that you have trust in them and that you value their insights a great deal. The same also applies when they come to you for your help and support in making decisions; it will make you feel loved and valued by them. This ultimately boosts your self-esteem and creates a more positive image of yourself. This is why having a supportive network of friends is essential so that you can influence one another and be there for each other when any of you really need it.

SAYING NO

None of us want to be the bad guy. None of us want to cause trouble or be difficult, particularly if there are expectations that we feel we have to meet no matter what. Whether it's a work email or a text from a friend, it feels perfectly natural to say yes at all times, even if the situation may be daunting and time consuming. After all, our entire lives have been molded over having a can-do attitude. But when was the last time that you said no to anyone?

Truth be told, we aren't doing ourselves any favors by constantly saying yes to everything. Even thinking about saying no can actually feel weird or even rude, and ultimately wrong. However, everyone has their limits and you are no exception. Saying no is an essential tool to help you create boundaries and manage expectations that others have of you, but we often overlook this tiny superpower that can actually work wonders for our mental health. Because of this, we find ourselves constantly working long hours or going to events that we have no interest in just because we are afraid of sounding impolite.

Therefore, saying no goes hand-in-hand with making time for the things that you love and helping you feel good about yourself. The more we say yes and avoid saying no, the harder we are making things for ourselves in the long run. And it all boils down to how saying no makes us actually feel—uncomfortable and awkward. Simply being put on the spot when we want to say no to a request instantly swells anxiety; we feel our heart pounding and our words stuck in our throats. While our gut is screaming at us to say no, we end up saying yes simply because it is the easy way out and keeps the other person happy and satisfied. But this is not actually creating any sort of balance as you put yourself at risk of being stressed out, overworked, and resentful.

Ultimately, there is no shame in saying no. You don't have to validate yourself or justify the reasons behind it. Only you are capable of doing the math on how much time and effort you have to put in for a certain request. You don't need a "good" reason to say no. It could be because of your personal preferences, existing priorities, scheduling conflicts, but it is not something that you need to explain in great detail. The final decision is yours, and it is one that you make after careful consideration.

That doesn't mean you start raising your hand to refuse every little thing. There are always going to be responsibilities that you have to take care of and say yes to, whether it is at home or work, or even your own health. The goal here is to be able to trust your intuition about something that you know perfectly well will be over-taxing for you, and make a mental reasoning over what you should do in all good conscience.

What exactly does saying no do for you, though? Tons of things. For starters, it makes you understand the value of your time and schedule, so you will value your "yeses" even more. If it is something that you love and enjoy doing, it is definitely worth saying yes to. This way, you will make time for things that add value to your life rather than take up your time unnecessarily. Furthermore, your yeses become more powerful and not just a passive answer to everything. You begin to stand up for yourself and say no to relationships and friendships that bring you grief, or extra assignments or projects that you know you cannot do efficiently and on time. You can also say no to people who want you to buy into their opinions or agree with things that stand in contrast to your beliefs.

Not just that, you should also learn to say no to yourself and listen when your inner voice tells you that you are about to make a bad decision. If you are thinking about getting yourself something you know you cannot afford, there has to be the inner voice that will tell you no, even if it hurts. Most of the time, you will have to push your desires aside and think of the long-term.

7

CHOOSE NATUROPATHIC MEDICINE

No matter how much you try, you will find that fighting the root causes of depression isn't a matter of taking a pill to make your problems go away. This is because the problems lie at the very heart of our beings as a result of the neuro-chemical processes our mind triggers in response to depression. No matter what the trauma, the anxiety level, the unique biology, or sensitivity of the person is, the standard medical protocol followed by doctors is to use antidepressants that will yield very few long-term results. This will continue to be the case until there is a detailed study of the patient's emotions and why they are the way they are. The need to understand why these emotions emerge to the forefront and impair the function of healthy and happy human beings is imperative, and blocking such emotions with antidepressants will not make them go away.

In most cases, taking regular antidepressants is simply repressing the problem without addressing the root of it. And taking medication is only one of several treatment options and should only be recommended when the stage of depression is severe. Therefore, it is essential to look towards a long-term and natural cure that will not harm your body and its complex internal processes. From what we have learned in the previous chapters, a holistic approach consisting of a healthy diet, exercise, social bonding, self-improvement, and getting essential nutrients is the key to treating your mind, body, and spirit.

Looking at it from the perspective of a long-term solution, nature provides us with several ready-made and easily available solutions that can help to revitalize us at an internal level. We have already had a detailed look at the benefits of grains and foods that can contribute to a healthy diet. However, nature has far more bounty ready for us in the form of herbs and other plants that can be made into teas and tinctures that are not only safe to use for everyone, but also help to genuinely build our resilience to depression a great deal better than their pharmaceutical counterparts.

Naturopathic medicine, or naturopathy, is a system of natural remedies and solutions that have existed for countless centuries. Every culture and civilization has had its own form of naturopathy that has relied on herbs and techniques such as exercise, massage, acupuncture, balanced nutrition, and so on, to alleviate all sorts of ailments and provide a better quality of life. And it continues to this day, with the most recent form of major naturopathic upheaval brought to the United States from Germany in the 1800s.

Naturopathy has two clear cardinal rules: Treat the whole person and treat with a therapeutic order. The latter could range from the least invasive or aggressive to the most invasive or aggressive. The strategies followed by naturopaths look at the mental, emotional, and physical aspects of a person to help their concerns. These strategies are far likelier to help than the never-ending barrage of antidepressants, which studies have shown to be no more effective than a placebo when it came to treating mild to moderate depression.

So if people do not get completely better from antidepressants, what exactly are they good for? Though the chemical ingredients of antidepressants are useful in altering the moods of people with severe depression, people with mild to moderate depression need to have more wholesome changes to their lifestyles. The effect of antidepressants to help them overcome a depressive episode is simply the placebo effect. This enables the mind to work its magic in treating depression rather than the medicine itself. Furthermore, antidepressants come with their own side effects that often lead patients to venture into the world of naturopathic medicine. These side effects could include nausea, weight gain, increased appetite, fatigue, drowsiness, insomnia, blurred vision, dry mouth, changes in sex drive, dizziness, agitation, anxiety, restlessness, and constipation.

THE NATUROPATHIC APPROACH TO TREATING DEPRESSION

Expanding upon the therapeutic order of the naturopathic approach, let's start with the least invasive or aggressive first. The first thing to look out for here are the obstacles to reducing the symptoms. More often than not, our depression is largely situation-based, ranging from problems related to work, family, friendships, relationships, negative outlooks, and so on. Any one of these situations could be toxic enough to cause depression. Some of these situations can be changed, while others can't. The best thing to do is to try behavioral therapy that can help to identify unhealthy or potentially self-destructive behaviors in order to alter them for our best interest.

Behavioral therapy can teach you better coping strategies in order to change your outlook and perception of the situations that cause depression. Moreover, natural therapies can also work best whether the patient is alone or if they are with someone who they resonate with greatly, like a naturopathic practitioner. Much like behavioral therapy and medication management, being facilitated by a person who you can instantly connect with and open up to about your concerns is an essential component on the road to recovery.

Aside from behavioral therapy, naturopathy recommends exercise to release the feel-good hormones dopamine and serotonin, as well as adrenaline, to help us achieve a rush of positivity and energy. It helps us to create a healthier body image for ourselves that prompts us to exercise even more, not to mention getting the benefits of the great outdoors such as fresh air and sunlight. In short, naturopathy is all about connecting with the Earth when it comes to your physical fitness as well as your diet. More emphasis on fresh fruits and vegetables as well as whole foods is recommended as opposed to food with more saturated fats, trans fat, and processed foods. There is certainly no better feeling than having food rich in nutrients, vitamins, and minerals in the long-term as opposed to having an unhealthy and greasy burger and fries combo meal.

A major component of naturopathy is herbal and botanical medicine, which has seen its use dating back several centuries. Western herbal medicine, which has its roots in European and North American historical practices, is one of the most common traditional systems of herbal medicines practiced among naturopaths. Such herbal medicine is preferred by an estimated 4 billion people worldwide. The emphasis is placed on treating the underlying causes of health problems (such as depression) and greatly improving the overall health of a patient.

There has been a great deal of investigation in the efficacy of individual herbal medicines for depression and anxiety. For example, chamomile has been found to significantly reduce the symptoms of anxiety without any adverse effects at higher doses. Other herbs such as echinacea were found to decrease anxiety over a period of three days, and gotu kola reduced anxiety as well as the intensity of a startle response by 26%. Another herb called passionflower was seen to significantly reduce the symptoms of anxiety in three clinical trials while kava also has very good evidence of clinical efficacy and low side effects.

Zinc plays a crucial role in enzymatic reactions in the body, being responsible for at least 100 such reactions. Because enzymes are what enable such reactions to take place, they will not work optimally if the body has a zinc deficiency. It is essential to have enough zinc to maintain and develop neurological networks as well as communication. It is also believed to be a necessary cofactor for neurotransmitter production and function, which establishes a link between zinc and depression.

Moreover, the system of biotherapeutic drainage is a form of biological medicine that combines herbs and minerals to work for specific systems and organs, such as your central nervous system, endocrine system, cardiovascular system, and so on. With origins from Germany, France, and Holland, biotherapeutic drainage has been around since the 1920s and seeks to optimize a specific internal system's functions and correct any issues. The way it works is by opening the emunctories or primary organs that release waste products, such as the kidneys, lungs, bowels, and even the skin. These waste products or toxins are excreted by exhaling carbon dioxide, urination, bowel movements, and sweating.

But there are two other primary emunctories that are often overlooked, and these are the liver and the emotions. You may be familiar with the liver's function to convert toxic substances into non-toxic ones in order to excrete them from the body safely. However, if the liver's functions are compromised then these toxins may not be efficiently converted into non-toxic substances, which can interfere with our health. Similarly, we also have a build-up of emotional toxins that also interfere with our well-being.

In the case that the primary emunctories are blocked from excreting their waste, the body attempts to excrete them through secondary emunctories such as the mucous membranes, musculoskeletal system, skin and mental/emotional processes. However, these systems are less efficient than the primary ones and our body shows obvious symptoms of a blockage in proper excretion such as chronic sinus or vaginal infections, benign prostatic hyperplasia (BPH), joint or muscle pain, skin rashes, infections, and depression. All of these are signs that the body is diverting toxic waste to the secondary emunctories and is taxing your overall health because it is not being done efficiently. This could lead to acute and chronic illnesses, chronic disease, and genetic weaknesses, as well as creating blockages to therapeutic treatment.

Biotherapeutic drainage aims to support and cleanse the blocked emunctories by a gentle elimination of toxins. Once this is achieved, it can allow you to achieve better health by balancing cell and organ function. It also activates enzymes and triggers immune function. Ultimately, this treatment helps to correct the pathology by correcting the physiology first in a thorough and easier manner.

Homeopathy is also a tried-and-tested method to correct mood disorders. Using natural ingredients instead of pharmaceutical ones, homeopathy provides similar benefits to biotherapeutic drainage, and can be considered as "green allopathy." Moreover, homeopathic medicines have little to no negative side effects that are a critical cause for concern among patients who are worried about potential interactions. They also don't interact with other medications, supplements, or herbs. The naturopath looks at a person's overall health, including their physical, mental, and emotional health, and attempts to match them to any of 5,000 remedies. This might appear to be a daunting task, but a talented naturopath is able to find the perfect remedy in a timely manner.

Let us examine the case of one male patient who was happily married for a year, but had started showing signs of fatigue, depression, anxiety, anger issues, and low libido. The problem wasn't his relationship as it was apparent that he was attracted to his wife. However, he stated that he had problems focusing and concentrating, as well as being unmotivated. Further probing also highlighted that they had moved from a sunny location to a place with frequent rain and a colder, darker environment. Aside from that, he had also had difficulties in gaining employment and making new friends.

His physician conducted the usual series of tests for natural causes such as iron-deficiency anemia, B vitamin–induced anemia, hypothyroidism, testosterone, low vitamin D, and low cholesterol. All the tests looked good with the exception of vitamin D, which was slightly low. The treatment lasted for six weeks with measures such as restoring vitamin D levels, adding Omega-3 supplements, and encouraging him to go out and look for friends and jobs rather than staying at home.

However, the patient did not see any changes in his demeanor so the doctor gave him a homeopathic remedy. But the patient emailed him to say that despite not having any suicidal thoughts, he was still not feeling well. This is a common stage in homeopathic treatment known as a healing crisis, which basically means that the symptoms would get worse before getting better. After getting a different homeopathic remedy, the patient experienced a huge change a month later, stating that he could concentrate properly and had also regained his passion for photography. Furthermore, he no longer needed the services of a counselor and had also seen an improvement in his marital relationship. A follow-up three months later showed that he still felt great after the treatment.

TYPES OF DEPRESSION

Feeling sad or low most of the time can affect your daily life and impair your regular functions. In such cases, you may actually have clinical depression and it can be treated by consulting a doctor or a therapist, taking medication, and making changes to your lifestyle. There are different types of depression which are caused either by different chemical changes in your brain or because of certain impactful and traumatic events in your life. Detailing how the depression is affecting you is a slow process which starts by talking to your doctor about your feelings and mental state. Based on some questions and getting further details about your life, a mental health specialist will be able to determine the type of depression you have. Diagnosing this is vital as it will help to decide the correct treatment plan for your condition.

The first is major depression, which may also be called a major depressive disorder. This is when you feel depressed most days of the week and for greater periods of time during the day. The obvious symptoms of a major depressive disorder are losing interest in activities that gave you pleasure, gaining or losing weight, having difficulty in sleeping or feeling sleepy during the day, feeling restless, agitated, and irritable, being sluggish or unmotivated due to having no energy, despondency, gloom or grief, unexplained aches and pains, having feelings of low self-worth or guilt over past decisions, and even being unable to make new decisions. Worst case scenario, you may even contemplate self-harm or suicide.

If you have five or more of these symptoms on most days for two weeks or longer, your mental health specialist may diagnose this as major depression. In any case, having a depressed mood or loss of interest in pleasurable activities must be at least one of these symptoms. The road to recovery could include therapeutic measures such as talk therapy where your mental health specialist will help you find ways to manage your depression. This may also include the use of antidepressants to alter your mood from a depressive state. However, there are other options when talking and medication do not work, such as electroconvulsive therapy (ECT), transcranial magnetic stimulation (TMS), and vagus nerve stimulation (VNS). All of these therapies stimulate certain areas of brain activities using different methods. ECT works with electrical pulses, TMS uses a special kind of magnet, and VNS uses an implanted device. The goal is to help the parts of the brain that control your mood in order to help them function better.

Following major depressive disorder is persistent depressive disorder, which normally lasts for two years or more. Previously it was known as low-grade persistent depression, or dysthymia and chronic major depression. Symptoms of persistent depressive disorder include not eating enough or overeating, not getting enough sleep or sleeping longer than necessary, fatigue, having low self-esteem or feelings of inadequacy, concentration and memory problems, problems at school or work, being indecisive, lack of joy, social withdrawal, and feeling hopeless. Treatment for persistent depressive disorder includes psychotherapy, medication, or a combination of the two.

Bipolar disorder, also known as manic depression, comprises mood episodes ranging from extremes such as having high energy and an upbeat mood to low and depressive periods characterized by symptoms of major depression listed earlier. The manic phase is characterized by having high energy, not getting enough sleep, racing thoughts and speech, being irritable, having grandiose thoughts, increased self-esteem and confidence, unusual, risky, or self-destructive behavior, and feelings of euphoria.

These mood swings can be curbed using medication. Doctors may suggest mood stabilizers such as lithium regardless of being in a high or low period. Currently, Seroquel, Latuda, and an Olanzapine-fluoxetine combination have been approved by the FDA to treat the depressed phases, though some doctors may recommend off-label medication, such as the anticonvulsant lamotrigine or the atypical antipsychotic Vraylar, for bipolar disorders.

Most conventional antidepressants are not always recommended to be used to treat bipolar disorder as a first option as studies have not provided sufficient evidence that they work as well as a placebo. Furthermore, traditional antidepressants run the risk of triggering a high phase of bipolar disorder in a small percentage of such patients, or they may increase the frequency of having more bipolar episodes over an extended period.

A frequently talked about one is psychotic depression which has the symptoms of major depression. However there are psychotic symptoms as well. These may include experiencing hallucinations (visual or auditory), having delusions, and being paranoid about anyone trying to harm you. These can be further expanded into different types such as delusions of grandeur, invincibility, or authority, and paranoia about being under threat from jealous co-workers, the government, or even aliens. These may be treated by a combination of antidepressant and antipsychotic medication, with ECT also being a viable option.

Two that are often confused are peripartum and postpartum depression. Peripartum depression can occur about four weeks before childbirth; postpartum depression can occur up to four weeks after. It is widely believed that it only happens to women giving birth, however, it could also happen to men after witnessing any such depression in their partners. Nearly one in ten men also experience it in the peripartum period. Women experiencing this could have symptoms related to bipolar disorder, postpartum psychosis, and thoughts of suicide. Other symptoms of peripartum and postpartum depression include anxiety, sadness, exhaustion, rage or anger, constantly worrying about the baby's health and safety, facing difficulties while caring for the baby, or even thoughts of self-harm or harming the baby.

Women may also experience premenstrual dysphoric disorder (PMDD) at the start of their period which is characterized by the symptoms of depression. Such symptoms include mood swings, anxiety or panic attacks, irritability, problems in concentration, fatigue, problems sleeping, feelings of being overwhelmed, changes in appetite, and so on. Much like peripartum and postpartum depression, PMDD is also believed to be linked to hormonal changes. Aside from antidepressants, oral contraceptives may sometimes be used to treat PMDD.

There are also other types of depression such as situational depression, where a stressful event could be impacting your overall mental health. This could be caused by events such as losing a job or being under financial strain. It could also come from problems in relationships such as physically abusive relationships that could lead to divorce, separation, and also child custody issues or extensive legal problems. Grief caused by a long-term illness in the family or even death of a loved one can cause situational depression. Symptoms of situational depression include sadness and hopelessness, frequent crying, anxiety, changes in appetite, problems with sleeping, aches and pains, lack of energy and fatigue, loss in concentration, and social withdrawal. Though it is not technically labeled as situational depression, most doctors refer to this as a stress response syndrome and it could be treated using psychotherapy.

On the other hand, there is also atypical depression that is considered to be a specifier describing a pattern of depressive symptoms. Symptoms of atypical depression include an increased appetite, a heavy feeling in your limbs, having a poor body image, being oversensitive to criticism and worrying about rejection, assorted aches and pains, and sleeping more than necessary. Atypical depression can be reduced by a positive event that could temporarily improve your mood, while antidepressants such as selective serotonin reuptake inhibitor (SSRI) or monoamine oxidase inhibitor (MAOI) could be recommended by a doctor.

And, of course, there is seasonal affective disorder (SAD) which we have covered extensively as a form of depression that usually occurs as a response to the long, cold, and gloomy days of the winter months. It is treated by getting as much sunlight as possible but light therapy for 15 to 20 minutes a day is also helpful. This should be considered as a first option instead of using antidepressants.

Oftentimes, vitamin supplements can be recommended to help manage depression and moods as well as other functions. People with low levels of B vitamins are more likely to face depression, particularly with low levels of vitamin B12. Our bodies may also find it difficult to absorb required amounts of vitamin B12 as we age, even without any particular disorder. Nevertheless, vitamin B12 can combat fatigue which is a symptom of depression.

Vitamin B12 is available in large concentrations in food such as fish, chicken, eggs, milk, and lean meats, as well as some breakfast cereals that are fortified with B12. Vegans or vegetarians who do not follow a meat-based diet might not be getting the required intake of vitamin B12, thus they may be advised to take supplements.

Aside from vitamin B12, there are other vitamins that could provide enrichment towards brain health such as vitamin B3. Also known as niacin, vitamin B3 helps with low levels of serotonin which can also contribute to depression among people. Lower levels of vitamin B3 lead to a negative mood and can also bring down the levels of serotonin with them. Therefore it is recommended to have a 20 mg dose of vitamin B3 daily to counteract the negative mood.

Vitamin B9 is usually advised for pregnant women as well as women who may want to have children at some stage. Not only can it help the synthesis of serotonin and thus with mood regulation, it can also help to lower brain-related birth defects during pregnancy. Vitamin B9 is also known as folic acid and folate.

Also, vitamin C supplements aid greatly with both mood regulation and cognitive function. Most people feeling fatigued or depressed have also been observed to have a vitamin C deficiency. Certain studies have shown an improvement in mood after taking vitamin C supplements among people with lower than normal levels. They have also been observed to reduce symptoms and levels of depression and anxiety in studies. Eating fruits and vegetables rich in vitamin C such as oranges and red peppers should provide you with an adequate supply. Aside from that, vitamin C supplements can be taken while staying in the upper limit of 2,000 mg a day.

Other natural vitamins such as Omega-3 fatty acids could help with depression, as they are essential for seamless brain function and health. These can be obtained from salmon and certain other fatty fish, as well as seeds and nuts. Magnesium is another ingredient for producing feel-good hormones in the brain which can stave off the symptoms of depression and other mood disorders. As per the medical journal Nutrition Reviews, some amount of magnesium deficiency is prevalent among nearly half of all adults in the United States. Aside from causing symptoms of depression, a magnesium deficiency can also lead to insomnia, muscle tension, and constipation.

USING BACH FLOWER REMEDIES

Another preferred naturopathic therapy is using Bach flower remedies. Created in the early 1900s by Edward Bach, a medical and homeopathic doctor, these remedies can be used as an alternative or complementary treatment for emotional problems and pain. According to Bach, the body could be healed by healing the negative emotions first. Based on his system, there are 38 different remedies that each address a specific negative emotion. These remedies are obtained from watered-down extracts of wild plant flowers as well as other minerals in a similar fashion to homeopathy. However, these remedies use fewer materials and target the specific emotions rather than the physical symptoms.

There are seven groups of broad psychological causes of illness: fear, uncertainty, lack of interest in present circumstances, loneliness, oversensitivity to influences and ideas, sadness or despair, and care for others at your own expense. Bach flower remedies do not really pose any side effects aside from a headache or rush. They may give the feeling of not wanting to take them regularly. This could be because you are forgetting them after your emotional state has returned to a proper balance. Another reason for not wanting to take them is because it may not be the right flower for your body in the present moment.

Some of the most commonly used Bach flower remedies include mustard for depression that comes and goes without any reason, and elm for whenever you feel overwhelmed, stressed out, or feel that you have too much to do in too little time that leads to depression. Pine can be used for feelings of guilt, particularly for things that are beyond your control or not your fault. Gentian is good for feelings of discouragement and failure that may arise from small setbacks. Cherry plum is for when you can sense you are about to lose control of your emotions or actions. Larch can help with feelings of low self-esteem, while hornbeam helps with feeling unable to cope with the day ahead of you. Such feelings can lead you to procrastinate and complain about things being too hard. Similarly, olive can help with lack of energy and exhaustion, and white chestnut can aid with having unwanted thoughts over and over again. Finally, aspen can help with feelings of oncoming dread, when you have a feeling that something bad is about to happen.

BENEFITS OF LAVENDER ESSENTIAL OIL

Plant-based treatments may also include the extracts of certain flowers such as lavender, which has been used for centuries as a treatment for depression. Lavender is a member of the Labiatae family and has been documented as an antibacterial, antifungal, anti-inflammatory, antiseptic, antimicrobial and carminative solution, as well as a sedative and antidepressant. It can also be used to help with eczema, nausea, and menstrual cramps, and could also have antispasmodic, analgesic, detoxifying, and hypotensive effects. Other uses for lavender are for cosmetic purposes as it is a mainstay variant of several personal care products.

Native to the Mediterranean, the Arabian Peninsula, Russia, and Africa, the most common species of lavender used for healthcare purposes is Lavandula angustifolia, also known as English Lavender. It can be used internally or by inhaling its essence. Lavender can be obtained as an essential oil or dried. It has a high concentration of volatile oils that create its unique and pleasurable scent which promotes relaxation. This fragrance has led to its use in aromatherapy to help with mild anxiety and exhaustion. Moreover, it can also be used internally for anxiety, insomnia, and gastrointestinal distress. Modern analysis has discovered that lavender oil contains more than 160 constituents, mainly linalool, linalyl acetate, terpinen-4-ol, and camphor. Most of these interact in a synergy that creates its therapeutic effects.

Studies have shown that lavender helps with anxiety thanks to its appealing scent. Physiology and Behavior published a study in 2005 that showed people waiting for dental treatment experienced decreased anxiety and improved mood just by breathing in a lavender scent. Another study has shown the benefits of aromatherapy with lavender oil in reducing anxiety among women with high-risk postpartum depression. Dietary supplements containing lavender oil could also have therapeutic effects for people with anxiety or stress.

Other studies show that lavender oil therapy, combined with better sleep hygiene techniques, could help in getting better sleep by inhaling lavender at bedtime. It also showed better energy and vibrancy after waking up the next day. While one study showed such results among college students, another found an improved quality of sleep and duration among an elderly population. Lavender oil stimulates a region of the brain known as the limbic system, which in turn helps to regulate emotions. This works both by breathing in the scent or applying lavender essential oil on the skin. It can also be blended with carrier oils such as jojoba or sweet almond, and then be used in baths or for massages.

Other methods include using a vaporizer or aromatherapy diffuser in the room to create the perfect mood for anyone, or even sprinkling some on a handkerchief to inhale it. However, be sure that it is pure lavender oil by checking the label for Lavandula angustifolia. It should also not be diluted with other oils such as fractionated coconut oil, jojoba oil, or sweet almond oil, as these cannot be used in diffusers.

Do keep in mind that lavender oil may cause side effects in some individuals including an allergic reaction or skin irritation, not to mention headaches, nausea, or vomiting. In such cases, it is recommended to discontinue its use.

CONCLUSION

Throughout these chapters, we have taken a journey covering all aspects of our lives that require the right kind of attention in order to make us complete and whole. While we depend on our social circle and environment to contribute towards our overall health and well-being, we can only expect that kind of care and empathy if we are ready to show it to ourselves first. Recognizing yourself as a unique, talented, and valuable individual in your own right is what will make you the integral piece to the jigsaw puzzle of life that is incomplete without you.

And it all starts with you, or more importantly, prioritizing yourself before giving to others. Of course, the feeling of being generous and helping someone in need can feel euphoric, but it should not come at the expense of your own happiness. Think about all the times you say yes or "I'd be delighted to," or "Sounds like a plan." How often do you just blurt out a response without taking the time to think about it? What if it cuts into your schedule or if you are simply a people pleaser who can't help but say yes? It just goes to show that we have internalized the concept of being a good friend, partner, employee, parent, or neighbor by always saying yes. But this can cause your life balance to get out of sync.

It's also perfectly natural to feel a little bit of guilt whenever you do say no, however it will actually help you to maintain your mental health in the long run. And far from actually being selfish, prioritizing your own needs and showing yourself some self-care is a profound act. After all, you won't be able to take care of others if you aren't taking care of yourself.

Now that you have all the tools you need, go out there and use them!

REFERENCES

Alo Moves. (n.d.). "7 Mindfulness Exercises for Self-love." Alo Moves. Retrieved June 7, 2021, from https://blog.alomoves.com/mindfulness/7-ways-to-start-practicing-self-love-right-now

Ash, M. (2014, February 11). "Naturopathic Treatment Strategies for Depression." Clinical Education. https://www.clinicaleducation.org/resources/reviews/naturopathic-treatment-strategies-for-depression/

Australian Government Department of Health. (2013). "Purposeful Activity – Hobbies." Head to Health. https://headtohealth.gov.au/meaningful-life/purposeful-activity/hobbies

Batson, J. (2011). "Stress Research." The American Institute of Stress. https://www.stress.org/stress-research

Bauer, B. A. (2017). "Can Vitamin C Boost Your Mood?" Mayo Clinic. https://www.mayoclinic.org/healthy-lifestyle/nutrition-and-healthy-eating/expert-answers/benefits-vitamin-c/faq-20058271

Bernstein, R. (2016, July 26). "The Mind and Mental Health: How Stress Affects the Brain." Touro University WorldWide. https://www.tuw.edu/health/how-stress-affects-the-brain/#:~:text=According%20to%20several%20studies%2C%20chronic

Bhandari, S. (2020, February 18). "Exercise and Depression: Endorphins, Reducing Stress, and More." WebMD. https://www.webmd.com/depression/guide/exercise-depression#:~:text=When%20you%20exercise%2C%20your%20body

Bruno, K. (2009, June 15). "Stress and Depression." WebMD. https://www.webmd.com/depression/features/stress-depression.

Bryan, M. (2019, January 14). "Sex Hormones in Meat and Dairy Products." News Medical. https://www.news-medical.net/health/Sex-Hormones-in-Meat-and-Dairy-Products.aspx#:~:text=Growth%20hormones%20are%20a%20central

Casteleijn, D., Steel, A., Bowman, D., Lauche, R., & Wardle, J. (2019, April 20). "A Naturalistic Study of Herbal Medicine for Self-reported Depression and/or Anxiety a Protocol." Integrative Medicine Research. https://www.sciencedirect.com/science/article/pii/S2213422019300150?via%3Dihub

"Christopher Reeve Quotes and Sayings." (n.d.). Wise Sayings. Retrieved June 13, 2021, from https://www.wisesayings.com/authors/christopher-reeve-quotes/

Coelho, P. (2014, March 5). "When You Say 'Yes' to Others, Make Sure You Are Not Saying 'No' to Yourself." Twitter. https://twitter.com/paulocoelho/status/441268849871454208?lang=en

Demirci, K., Akgönül, M., & Akpinar, A. (2015). "Relationship of Smartphone Use Severity with Sleep Quality, Depression, and Anxiety in University Students." Journal of Behavioral Addictions, 4(2), 85–92. https://doi.org/10.1556/2006.4.2015.010

DeNoon, D. J. (2008, May 22). "Types of Depression." WebMD. https://www.webmd.com/depression/guide/depression-types

DiLonardo, M. J. (2019, January 29). "Bach Flower Remedies: Uses, Effectiveness, Side-Effects. WebMD. https://www.webmd.com/vitamins-and-supplements/bach-flower-remedies

Edermaniger, L. (2020, July 3). "9 Facts on Gut Bacteria and Mental Health, Probiotics and Depression." Atlas Biomed. https://atlasbiomed.com/blog/9-ways-gut-bacteria-and-mental-health-probiotics-and-depression-are-linked/

Faculty of Sports and Exercise Medicine UK. (n.d.). "The Role of Physical Activity and Sport in Mental Health." The Faculty of Sport and Exercise Medicine. https://www.fsem.ac.uk/position_statement/the-role-of-physical-activity-and-sport-in-mental-health/#:~:text=Physical%20activi-ty%20has%20been%20shown

"Five Health Benefits of Spending Time with Friends and Family." Road to Heaven Game. (2018, July 24). https://roadtoheavengame.com/health-benefits-spending-time-friends-and-family/

Foods, D. M. (2020, January 30). "1 in 3 Americans Say They Were Never Educated on Healthy Eating Habits." Cision PR Newswire. https://www.prnewswire.com/news-releases/1-in-3-americans-say-they-were-never-educated-on-healthy-eating-habits-300995996.html

"Getting Closer." Regina Mundi Catholic College. (n.d.). https://rmc.ldcsb.ca/apps/news/article/819575

Hall, D. (2017). "Can Chronic Stress Cause Depression?" Mayo Clinic. https://www.mayoclinic.org/healthy-lifestyle/stress-management/expert-answers/stress/faq-20058233

Harvard Health Publishing. (2018, August 1). "How Meditation Helps with Depression." Harvard Health. https://www.health.harvard.edu/mind-and-mood/how-meditation-helps-with-depression

Ieso Digital Health. (2021, May 10). "Mental Health Awareness Week: Relationships with Friends." Ieso Digital Health. https://www.iesohealth.com/en-gb/blog/mental-health-awareness-week-relationships-with-friends#:~:text=Having%20friends%20that%20we%20enjoy

"The Importance of Vitamin D to Your Happiness and Health." R3Bilt Fitness. (2020, June 24). http://r3bilt.com/2020/06/20/the-importance-of-vitamin-d/

King, C. (n.d.) "Biotherapeutic Drainage." Dr. Cheri King. Retrieved June 7, 2021, from https://www.drcheriking.com/about/biotherapeutic-drainage

Kryder, C., Godwin, J., & Oura-Admin. (2021, June 2). "Circadian Rhythms and Your Bedtime." The Pulse Blog. https://ouraring.com/blog/circadian-rhythms-bedtime/

Link, R. (2018, January 7). "11 Signs and Symptoms of Too Much Stress." Healthline. https://www.healthline.com/nutrition/symptoms-of-stress#TOC_TITLE_HDR_2

Lustig, R. (2018, April 15). "Big Food and Big Pharma: Killing for Profit." Robert Lustig. https://robertlustig.com/2018/04/malhotra-eu-big-food-pharma/

McCabe, C. (2021, February 12). "The Science Behind Why Hobbies Can Improve Our Mental Health." The Conversation. https://theconversation.com/the-science-behind-why-hobbies-can-improve-our-mental-health-153828

Melinda. (2021, June 14). "Stress Symptoms, Signs, and Causes." HelpGuide. https://www.helpguide.org/articles/stress/stress-symptoms-signs-and-causes.htm#:~:text=Chronic%20street%20

Mendelsohn, P. (2019, July 26). "The Importance of Saying 'No'." myTherapyNYC. https://mytherapynyc.com/importance-of-saying-no/

Monroe, J. (2018, April 3). "Teens and Sports: The Exercise–Mental Health Link." Newport Academy. https://www.newportacademy.com/resources/mental-health/sports-and-mental-health/

Mosier, L. (2016, February 1). "The Power of Saying No." Wanderlust. https://wanderlust.com/it/journal/the-power-of-saying-no/#:~:text=Saying%20no%20-gives%20your%20yes

Nall, R. (2019, November 12). "Stress and Constipation: What Is the Link?" Medical News Today. https://www.medicalnewstoday.com/articles/326970#:~:text=High%20levels%20of%20stress%20can

Nittle, N. (2020, December 29). "Vitamin D Deficiency and Depression: What's the Connection?" Verywell Mind. https://www.verywellmind.com/the-link-between-vitamin-d-and-depression-5089428

Practical Psychology. (2020, March 21). "Fight or Flight (The Adrenal Response)." Practical Psychology. https://practicalpie.com/fight-or-flight/

Raypole, C. (2020, January 29). "Meditation for Depression: Why It Works and How To Start." Healthline. https://www.healthline.com/health/meditation-for-depression#benefits

Robinson, L., Segal, J., & Smith, M. (2019, June). "The Mental Health Benefits of Exercise: The Exercise Prescription for Depression, Anxiety, and Stress." Helpguide. https://www.helpguide.org/articles/healthy-living/the-mental-health-benefits-of-exercise.htm

Rodger, A. (1970, January 1). "Whistle-Binkie; A Collection of Songs for the Social Circle. Series 1-4: Rodger, Alexander, 1784-1846." Internet Archive. https://archive.org/details/whistlebinkieco00carruoft/page/n297/mode/2up?view=theater

Rosenberg, M. (2017, September 24). "How Big Pharma and Big Food Have Made Us Fat and Sick." Salon. https://www.salon.com/2017/09/24/how-big-pharma-and-big-food-have-made-us-fat-and-sick_partner/

Smith, R. (2004). "Let Food Be Thy Medicine..." British Medical Journal. https://www.ncbi.nlm.nih.gov/pmc/articles/PMC318470/#:~:text=Mark%20Lu-cock%20ends%20his%20review

"Stress: A Social Issue." Brunet. (2019). https://www.brunet.ca/en/health/health-tips/le-stress--un-enjeu-de-societe/

Suni, E. (2020, November 3). "Light and Sleep: Effects On Sleep Quality." Sleep Foundation. https://www.sleepfoundation.org/bedroom-environment/light-and-sleep

"Symptoms of Depression." The Original Bach Flower Remedies. (2012, November 6). http://www.bachflower.com/symptoms-of-depression/

Tolle, E. (1999). The Power of Now: A Guide to Spiritual Enlightenment. New World Library.

"Vitamins That Help With Depression." The Recovery Village Drug and Alcohol Rehab. (2019, February 13). https://www.therecoveryvillage.com/mental-health/depression/related/vitamins-for-depression/

"Wee Willie Winkie | Nursery Rhymes and Traditional Poems." Lit2Go. (n.d.). https://etc.usf.edu/lit2go/74/nursery-rhymes-and-traditional-poems/5373/wee-willie-winkie/

"Why It's Time to Ditch the Phone Before Bed." SCL Health (2018). https://www.sclhealth.org/blog/2019/09/why-it-is-time-to-ditch-the-phone-before-bed/

Witkamp, R. F., & Norren, K. van. (2018, June 21). "Let Thy Food Be Thy Medicine....When Possible." European Journal of Pharmacology. https://www.sciencedirect.com/science/article/pii/S0014299918303595?via%3Dihub

Wong, C. (2016). "The Health Benefits of Lavender Essential Oil." Verywell Mind. https://www.verywellmind.com/lavender-for-less-anxiety-3571767

Yang, L., Zhao, Y., Wang, Y., Liu, L., Zhang, X., Li, B., & Cui, R. (2015). "The Effects of Psychological Stress on Depression." Current Neuropharmacology. 13(4),

494–504. https://doi.org/10.2174/1570159x1304150831150507

Zelman, K. M. (2011, June 21). "Tips for Reaping the Benefits of Whole Grains." WebMD. https://www.webmd.com/food-recipes/features/reap-the-benefits-of-whole-grains#:~:text=Whole%20grains%20are%20packed%20with

Printed in Great Britain
by Amazon

28339811R00089